A Sensory Approach to Improving Muscle Control

A Sensory Approach to Improving Muscle Control

An Engineer's View On Optimal Fitness

Martin L. Vanderhook

To order additional copies of this book, contact:
Xlibris Corporation
1-888-795-4274
www.Xlibris.com
Orders@Xlibris.com
63982

Contents

Prologue

"And while a scientist in the lab sees the laws of nature as the constraints by which he or she is bound, to an engineer in the field those same restrictions may be viewed as the obstacles which must somehow be overcome."

The aforementioned quote then being my very concise way of explaining why this book was written from the perspective of an engineer rather than a scientist, which would have been more correct. For in dealing with the intangible nature of our mental faculties my rather unconventional approach gives me the latitude to make certain presumptions that, due to their very rudimentary nature, may not exactly conform with what is generally acknowledged. Which is to say the descriptions expounding on our mental faculties are not as stringent as a scientific detailing would call for, since their purpose is not to define doctrine but merely to develop a more encompassing utilization of a normally mundane physical activity. However because of depicting things from an engineer's perspective an understanding of at least high school physics and chemistry, although not essential, helps to make my already simplistic interpretations less confounding.

I sense though that the actual technique described in this book will only be perused by a select few, as the ideas conveyed require not only a certain level of understanding but also an open-mindedness that, in today's world, seems a rare commodity. Hopefully though my explanations are not so abstract as to mystify even that rather diverse group of free thinkers. But enough about my personal reservations and on with a more prevailing belief that, in accordance with a new century, a more enlightened view should be taken about all the wondrous things we are able to experience and not just the various aspects as related to fitness, which I am about to address.

The Physical Mind and Introduction

Now from judging simply the generalized behavior of most young children I have encountered it would seem that almost everyone is born with an inquisitive nature. As time passes however while still awed by the appearance of a rainbow, from inquires I have made, a majority of adults questioned were no longer interested in what actually causes these illusionary arcs of color. I on the other hand, from having endured an upbringing of unadorned nurturing, still retain my curiosity for not only the more conspicuous wonders of creation, such as light dispersion through water vapor, but also other less obvious and sometimes more perplexing phenomena. In particular, for over twenty years, I have been intrigued by a most puzzling aspect of nature that although seemingly accessible is not readily evident, consequently making the concept of its existence a more dubious proposition.

The mysterious marvel to which I refer is of course none other than the engendering of our mental faculties into a seemingly a separate entity, denoted very simply as our mind. For although neurons have been identified as the essential component, defining the physical make-up of a human brain, a great deal of speculation still exists about what exactly results from the multitude of interconnections, whose scheme of interfacing is here defined in terms of the two extremes in our utilization. Where in an isolated sense, from a variety of testing, it has been established that what essentially underlies our ability to learn is how readily we are able to integrate what we experience. In terms of defining the culmination however of all neural activity our understanding is a bit more constrained with the output from some sort of monitoring device being really the only way we have been able to denote (in a very tangible sense) a conscious mind, from one lacking that rather unique feature. And so because of the lack of a definitive interpretation on the exact nature of the relationship between structure and function, at the highest level of convolution, is the reason as I see it for the discipline of psychology being defined by a variety of operational theories. Where initially rather than a more conventional reduction to a series of mathematical equations instead, at the onset of the last century, the behavior of another animal was used as a reference standard for making certain presumptions about our decision making process or essentially how our mind operates. In general though any conclusion reached, from studying the demeanor of a canine, was subject to more latitude of interpretation, compared to fields of study where results are construed through strictly numerical reasoning.

Today however for emulating a particular mode of evaluation, by the rather extensive area of our brain where all high-level or abstract information processing takes place, even psychology has been extended to encompass a more numerically based scheme, in its effort to better define the extent our mental faculties. With the actual driving force, behind this encroaching by psychology, being the sheer processing power of today's personal computer. Because although on a rudimentary level only able to compare ones and zeros it is from the unimaginably fast internal clock, the gating mechanism of every digital computer, that allows it to run a variety of software of such a degree of sophistication, as to actually surpass most of us at its intended task. The exception being when it comes to replicating certain inherent methods of processing sensory information, such as verbal communication, where due in part to the sheer number of variables involved reducing everything to simple code has been a more perplexing task. And so innovative programmers, as a way to improve on linguistics decoding, have in part gone to the source by creating virtual constructs, analogous to the actual neural networking of our brain. For the prevailing theory on the processing of sensory information, by the gray matter within our cranium, is based on the interaction between a multitude of what are construed as intricately wired structural configurations, defined in a singular sense as simply a specific neural network. In effect alluding that way we think, albeit oftentimes also singular in nature, is a manifestation from analysis by a vast array of operationally discrete entities and not just a single integrated sensory information processor, but more on that later.

So what intrigues me about the human brain (and mine in particular) is that normally while awake, through an almost distinct discerning of my own consciousness, I sense or at least seem to sense a kind of physical presence to my mind. If I lose consciousness however, such as when falling asleep, my brain's reduced neural activity no longer sustains my sense of self-awareness and so seemingly my mind has ceased to exist, although physically nothing appears to have changed. An analogy to this dilemma, on the substance of our mind, can be seen in the early study of electricity where voltage was the only parameter for defining the transfer of electrons between two separated carbon rods, even though the transition is also denoted by an arc of light. For while the generated flash of electromagnetic radiation was easily sensed, through mere observation, it could only be referenced through arbitrarily comparing its intensity. Because unlike with voltage where, through the intermediary of an associated magnetic field, there was some sort of basis for a set electrical charge defining a certain mechanical force, light was yet to be correlated with any known standards. For not only was there an "ether" issue, which related to transmission, since there was also the fundamental conundrum whereby, depending on how it was viewed, the behavior of light could reflect the dynamics of either a wave or a particle. And although other questions were raised the ether dilemma was resolved after the Michelson-Morley experiment established that, unlike with sound, light gives no indication of being necessarily associated with a conducting medium. The central issue however, defining the exact nature of light, required such a novel interpretation that it was to initially establish the foundation of a seemingly abstract branch of physics, whose revelations have actually impacted on all fields of scientific inquiry. For our incorporating of the enigmatic principles of quantum mechanics has meant that, once a cornerstone of science, the allusion of absolute certainty had to be amended with the reality that only a certain degree of probability dictates if a stated event will occur. And so we begin a new millennium with science also having a way to effectively assess the "spark" denoting an active mind, although adequately defining the resulting "light" is still an issue of considerable debate.

Now before being intrigued by the workings of the human brain, through engaging in some form of fitness conditioning, my curious nature had been directed primarily at extending my physical potential, either in terms of strength or stamina. The underlying reason though I feel, for such a high degree of self-interest, is because a compelling attribute of my inquisitive demeanor has turned out to be a striving for efficiency, possibly brought on by the pervasive influence of my father being a manager by profession. Where initially at the age of sixteen this optimizing approach to life is what led to an assessing that, to improve on the maturation process affecting me, I should take up weightlifting. Although on the inside cover of most comic books I had read, just a few years earlier, that is also what the Charles Atlas ads seemed to imply. And so for almost a full two years, leading up to my entry into military service, I for the most part adhered to a rather extensive weightlifting routine, which effectively engaged all pertinent sets of skeletal musculature.

Now after completing the initial phase of my obligation, although time and availability were not an issue, it was just not in me to go back to my old routine of resistance conditioning. Less than two years would pass however before, although my activity of choice now being running, I was once again actively involved in the extending of my physical endowment. The reason though for this change, in my approach to staying in shape, was because my insatiable thirst for understanding had uncovered that, since its effect is ultimately felt throughout our body, aerobic conditioning should really be developed before or in conjunction with a program of resistance-conditioning exercises. Because with almost every approach to overload conditioning, from following the prescribed routine, the impact of the physical stress incurred is generally localized to just the specific muscle groups and support systems actually employed. The exception being any circuit-type program where a series of resistance-conditioning exercises are done as per standard practice but with little or no rest permitted between sets, which is normally a concession. A lack of respite is then used to keep one's heart rate elevated for the extended period of time needed to affect the various physiological adaptations, most noticeably perceived through an increase in physical stamina.

The preceding explanation I believe was originally conveyed to me by *The Complete Book of Running* which in nineteen seventy-eight was the reference source that initially established my approach to just running, although the various conditioning alternatives (discussed throughout the book) could be applied to a number of physical activities. Four years later, in nineteen eighty-two, is when my interest in personal development was suddenly extended to encompass my mental faculties, after having read the book *Brain Power 'Learn To Improve Your Thinking Skills'*. For I was so intrigued by the author's analysis of this process we call thinking that anything published, on topics ranging from how the brain functions to the fundamentals of artificial intelligence, was now subject to my unrelenting curiosity.

It was then from being exposed, to such a variety of interpretations, that I gained a fuller understanding of how our concept of reality encompasses not only what is "out there". For our perception of our environment is in fact a fabrication of our brain built on not just sensory information from our five senses, as our notion of reality is also influenced by the information already encoded in our memory. Because without an ability to summarize and retain everyday occurrences the processing of any sensory information would be like continually experiencing it for the first time. But through correlating with a built-up neural database, which gives meaning to what we perceive, previously identified information patterns are oftentimes processed on a pre-conscious level and so any unknown stimuli, initially detected as a possible threat, can be quickly attended to by our consciousness. If however, as a rather extreme example, that "threat" turned out to be simply an inability to readily recollect the specific features that characterize a ball, being hurled in our direction. What would compel us to try and better integrate the essential attributes of any ball, depicted initially in a similar fashion as simply a circle enclosing a spherical color scheme?

Simple curiosity of course as it initially inspires most of us at an early age to seek out not only the name of every object we happen come across. For oftentimes our curious nature compels us to try and develop an even more detailed series of memories that convey physical properties, such as most balls can be rolled but only some will bounce. Leading to the contention that, early in life, our inherent inquisitiveness is based on simply a need to create a neural database of sufficient complexity, for navigating the particular environment in which we are raised. From my rather limited perspective however, as an observer of human behavior, it seems that for many this innate thirst for knowledge tends to wane and turn superficial, after achieving not much more than a rudimentary level of understanding. Hopefully though the underlying cause, for this apparent trivializing of our inherent curiosity, is more from a lack of nurturing, rather than a reflection of innate programming.

But from merely a personal assessment I would like to extend this line of speculation to encompass the specific structural configuration, whose neural processing actually embodies the essence of mental faculties. And so based on just physical appearance it would appear that this neural plexus, which also defines the source of our sense of self-awareness, is not confined to a central location but encompasses a cerebral cortex consisting of a distinct left and right hemispheric lobe. With the contention being that, as a result of being rent asunder, we functionally have (connected by a corpus callosum) not one but two separate areas that rather independently analyze sensory information, thus defining the two-brain theory. On a conscious level however the actual disparity in processing, by each hemispheric lobe, would be denoted through an evoking of two different interpretations, based on discerning different aspects of an incurred stimulus. But although perceptual dichotomy may be applied to each sense normally it is most evident as related to visual processing by our sense of sight and not our sense of touch, on which muscle control is based. My example of bilateral sensory information processing, as expressed through a subtle distinction in our visual perception, is even elegantly stated in the phrase "seeing the trees from the forest". For we can literally make a conscious decision to seemingly alter our perceived view, from an undefined emphasis on the forest and its surroundings, to intently gazing at just a single or a set number of trees.

Of course in terms of physiology this subtle difference in our visual perspective, between surveying and scrutinizing, is alluded to as being merely a reflection of a slight shift in focus by our eyes. However when defined in terms of sensory information processing the variance in our mental projection, between an overview of the forest and intently gazing at a few individual members, is more profound than can be explained through simply our eye muscles working to deform a set of lenses. The presumption though of our having distinct centers of sensory evaluation allows this disparity in our visual perspective, between surveying and scrutinizing, to be denoted by our decision to primarily engage either our left or right cerebral cortex, depending on our intent. But before further discussing the two-brain theory, stipulating a difference in the bilateral processing of sensory information, the design and function of a neuron will first be considered.

Now as the actual component whose mere filtering of signal transmission, to inhibit or facilitate, is what underlies any thought process we are said to engage in that means besides our brain a neuron is also the defining building block, whose level of interfacing essentially establishes the viability our mind. A neuron then, as the discrete element employed in the processing of sensory information, is analogous to a gate, the most rudimentary electrical circuit used for manipulating digital information. And as each is designed to trigger a single output, usually initiated through the precise timing from any number of input signals, that means functionally a neuron and an electronic gate are also very similar. The difference then, between neural tissue and most digital circuits, is in the discriminating process each one actually employs. For although timing is crucial to the operation of both types of discerning with digital processing the use of voltage levels is rather crude as variations in a set state of information (either a one or a zero) can oftentimes be quite significant. With neural tissue, on the other hand, the situation is more exacting because neurons are not only more precise but are also oftentimes more versatile in being able to be reprogrammed, through affecting the inherent impedance to triggering an output.

Irrespective though of the aforementioned operational difference a correlation can also be made between a set structure of neurons, defined in its most complex form as our brain, and a number of integrated electronic components, manifested at the highest level of convolution as a digital computer. The comparison here being applicable in the sense that the number of components each set structure is made-up of and the degree of integration, each discriminating element is subject to, are the same two factors defining the difference in the complexity of function between neural tissue and a digital circuit. Whereby on a wafer of silicon, "sprinkled" with some type of impurity, a central processing unit or CPU consists of nothing more than a large collection of gates, whose structure was originally formulated out of a number of Boolean Algebra equations. And so within our brain an apparently nondescript "clump" of neurons, whose interconnections were initially choreographed by evolution, can be likened to a sensory information processor. The cerebral cortex, residing within the protective casing of our skull, is then envisioned operationally as not just a single neural computer but as an integrated array, consisting of a significant number of relatively discrete structures for processing sensory information. But although functionally defined as an orchestration of interfacing our cerebrum in fact more closely resembles a chaotic aggregation, where any actual discerning of a specific neural network is almost impossible. However it is through the sensory information processing by the various neural networks, within the constraints of our cranium, that we are able to depict an intricate picture of our visual reality, from just the light painting the back of our eyes.

At birth however most of the neural networking, which defines a baby's brain, is not yet fully developed, hence the actual physiological basis to our inherent curiosity. And so from a variety of learning activities changes are reflected, within our brain, not only through neural reprogramming of resetting the initiating level to trigger an output but also by reconfiguring on a more permanent basis through the physical growth of new interconnections and/or the deactivating of neural links no longer being used. With of course the outpouring of sensory stimuli, from ideally all five senses, being a primary factor defining how the gray matter within our cranium actually goes about reorganizing itself, as a huge database for storing sensory information. Because any kind of impairment, to any one of our senses, would tend to affect a decrease in the processing of any related sensory stimuli, by the associated area of our brain. Oftentimes though we are able to invoke an encroaching, by a working sense, on the relatively underused part of our brain, which was previously employed in processing sensory stimuli from our damaged sense. The insinuation here being that, unlike with electronic circuitry, the physical structure of our brain is not a fixed commodity. For the neural networking, contained within our cranium, is thought to be rather malleable where changes are in part determined by the expanding of our mental faculties, through acquiring a new skill, or by allowing a diminishing in capacity to occur, through not maintaining a level of proficiency. Similar in principle to what has been more superficially applied to just our skeletal muscles, where you lose'um if you don't use'um.

As compelled by genetic programming however, with a normal human brain, there is a defined region explicitly designed for just processing the electrochemical signals, initially transduced from a very narrow bandwidth of electromagnetic radiation striking the back of our eyes. That area, where visual "reconstructing" first takes place, is of course the occipital lobe located at the back of our brain. The details however have not yet been fully uncovered on exactly how this particular region, defining the epicenter of our visual processing, actually interacts (with the rest of our brain) to create a seemingly unbroken spatial representation of our external surroundings. Nonetheless I have aspired to extend on a previous appraisal on the assessing of sensory stimuli by our brain, albeit largely based on conjecture. Where through an analogous comparison the aforementioned contrast in our visual perspective, between "surveying" and "scrutinizing", is seen as the difference between an analysis (of the electrochemical signals representing sensory stimuli) in a simultaneous fashion or a manner more sequential in nature. Which is to say the neural networking of our right cerebral cortex is envisioned as being configured primarily around a parallel or simultaneous processing of many different "bits", discerned from the overall electrochemical information pattern. While the left hemispheric lobe of our cerebrum is seen as being geared more towards an in-depth serial analysis of a single bit at a time. (A "bit" in this case being a simple metaphor for what is actually envisioned as a variable amount of sensory information; ranging in size from all the detail in a single integrated element, such as a tree, to encompassing merely a particular attribute, such as the shape or color of its leaves.) And so as consciously reflected through a slight shift, in the extent of our field of vision, now to briefly elaborate on the difference between a surveying and a scrutinizing perspective, as it relates to the processing of visual sensory information by each hemispheric lobe of our cerebrum.

As already noted then visual sensory information is initially transduced from electromagnetic radiation that, within the frequency bandwidth of visible light, encompasses the color spectrum of a rainbow. And so after being focused, by a lens in front, any direct or reflected light transitions to the back of each eye where, by a large number of frequency sensitive cones and rods, it is encoded into a series of electrochemical signals. Next in conjunction with our occipital lobe a rudimentary "reassembling" is achieved through forming or creating an initial visual representation, based on just "crude" bits of sensory information. With the color (derived from a specific frequency bandwidth) and the edges on and around an object (derived from the difference between two colors) being the two prime examples of this unrefined sensory information. Finally to try and affect a degree of comprehension, from the back of our brain, "crudely" reconstructed visual sensory information patterns are "conveyed" forward to be more precisely defined through referencing by both our left and right cerebrum, with the hemisphere of greatest activity indicating which interpretation predominates. The phrase "surveying the forest" then implies that, since there is no specific item attracting our attention, our sense of awareness is being influenced more strongly by the operational parameters of our right cerebral cortex. Because the complete light radiation pattern, projected onto our occipital lobe, is in effect "disseminated" into a number of individual constructs, with the right hemispheric lobe of our cerebrum. Next by referencing to what is stored in our vast virtual database of memories these "detached" representations (of a particular element or merely a related attribute) are then readily identified, depending on what is being surveyed. Ultimately however the full impact, from successfully identifying most of the items we perceive, is that it allows for a more detailed view of our visual reality, even though we are no longer acutely discerning any of the particulars in our field of vision. But although a very complex and demanding task for our mental faculties this virtual deconstructing of what we visually perceive is however just one form of sensory information processing, by the right hemispheric lobe of our brain. Because when engaged in endeavors of a cognitive nature our right cerebrum is also the source of our intuition, where analysis is not based on deductive reasoning (the mode of processing our left cerebral cortex was designed for).

And so when something does enter our field of vision, which is not readily identified, we will usually tend to affect a coalescing of our surveying perspective, by our right cerebrum, into an intent focus by the left hemispheric lobe of our bilateral brain. This then being when our eyes are compelled into selectively scanning, within a defined area of space, the various characteristics such as color, texture and shape of oftentimes a single construct. And so this acute discerning, by our left cerebrum, is then what essentially updates our mental database on what is being viewed. The enduring effect however, from the sequential analysis by our left cerebral cortex, is that it gives us the illusion of perceiving a more exacting depiction of anything previously scrutinized, even though it is no longer being observed directly. And with the corresponding alternative, to our visual dissecting of the object of our attention, being through a simultaneous comparing of its different features; in theory how the right cerebrum of our brain would discern just a single construct, from within our field of vision.

Obviously what has just been proposed is an overly simplified explanation of an ability we seemingly have to alter our field of vision, although not through a shift in focus by our eyes. Because where the emphasis resides in our utilization, by either our left or our right cerebral cortex, is what in theory defines the difference in our perspective, between indiscriminately surveying and intently gazing. Of course it may be questionable whether there is any real basis to sensory information actually being processed in the manner depicted, although what we know about the human brain is still rather superficial. But despite that limitation of lacking any definitive evidence my mere defining of a conceivable interface, between the two main lobes of our cerebrum, does expose a most intriguing aspect, related to the whole idea of bilateral sensory information processing. And that is the way I, through the detached scrutiny of my sense of self-awareness, can actually ascertain this subtle difference in the extent of my field of vision, between indiscriminately surveying and intently gazing. So what is this seemingly detached perspective, described as simply self-awareness, that allows me to discern an attribute of the first intangible of mere conscious awareness, the entity manifested from just the rudimentary processing of sensory information?

Well my understanding is that self-awareness is simply the realization of our brain, through a variety of learning activities, overcoming a certain threshold in progressively increasing neural integration. For any human brain, regardless of its size, is normally comprised of such a tremendous number of neurons that the possibilities for significantly extending on neural complexity are fundamentally established. Leading to the contention that self-awareness is acquired through merely "fine-tuning" the degree of interconnection already developed between the convoluted interweaving of neural circuitry, which gives our brain its outward physical appearance.

Now compared to mere awareness, our most rudimentary form of consciousness, self-awareness can be loosely defined as a more detached perspective with a much higher level of cognizance. Of course just analyzing a particular circumstance with an increased degree of insight doesn't necessarily validate any of the conclusions reached, mainly due our own prejudice or ignorance. Although any augmenting in the extent of our conscious perception usually allows for a more thorough understanding of a prevailing situation to make some kind of determination, compared to relying on simply instinctive behavior. Under extreme duress however no matter how evolved our sense of self-awareness we are oftentimes reduced to reacting in an instinctive manner, resorting to our most basic response of either fight or flight.

Initially then, as defined by a degree of self-awareness, our ancestors primary use for a more detached or higher level of information processing was to develop social interaction skills, as that increased the probability of genetic survival. Additionally however, like us, early man was also endowed with an inherent curiosity and two very versatile appendages, our hands, that occasionally led him (or her) to fixate on other things, beyond just satisfying an emotional drive or a social need. As eventually this potent combination of both physical and mental dexterity is what enabled the inhabitants of certain early civilizations to develop some form of symbolic logic, the underlying basis to mathematics (the essential "tool" of technology that would in time allow for all the possibilities in today's high-tech world).

It was however after an extended introduction, lasting well into fifteenth century, before numerical reasoning started becoming increasingly more diverse as its implementation, as a methodology, was gradually expanded by a suddenly fervent quest to try and understand all the mechanisms of nature. That of course being the enlightened age of the Renaissance when, along with many other revelations, mathematics was finally acknowledged (throughout Europe) as the language of science, since a number of earlier civilizations had already made that determination. What that meant though (with the incorporation of mathematics) was to now gain recognition, as a scientific explanation, descriptions on the nature of phenomena had to be presented in such a way that just one or a whole series of numerical expressions were the only means employed, for predicting the outcome of a stated occurrence. And lasting until the onset of the twentieth century the impression given, by the underlying principles of physics, was that to a certain degree nature could be confined to the realm of absolute certainty, as postulated by the laws of Newtonian mechanics. So pervasive was this belief, in the power of numerical reasoning, that it seduced some scientists into envisioning the possibility of prophesying about the future, if only all the relevant variables could be determined. Interest quickly faded however when, during the early part of the last century, the acceptance of quantum mechanics and the extent of its impact effectively turned every event into a question of probability, forever eclipsing the notion of a clockwork universe.

Similar then to with earlier studies, seeking to define the exact nature of light, the deficiency of an encompassing numerical elucidation is also what confronts any research, trying to establish the basis for denoting our sense of self-awareness as being a distinct entity. Even more disconcerting however is that unlike with quantum mechanics, which essentially afforded a resolution by allowing for the possibility of two competing sets of equations to describe the behavior of light. Beyond rudimentary mimicry of our brain's neural networking research on the essence of the human mind has yet to give rise to any kind of viable construct, based on strictly numerical reasoning. Which is why, as defined by a sense of self-awareness, our consciousness still struggles, in terms of strictly empirical science, to achieve some type of recognition beyond being merely quantified either through directly measuring electrical activity, from individual sensors, or by indirectly correlating neural activity to blood flow.

On the other hand, as the embodiment of our mind, our sense of self-awareness is in some religions seen as being tantamount to the soul of a person and with the quest to achieve a more complete or ultimate sense self-awareness, a common life-long goal. This notion of there being varying degrees of self-awareness is even alluded to in psychology where the apex of consciousness is referred to as self-actualization. So even if empirical science has yet to establish the mere possibility of an adequate representation, based on strictly numerical reasoning, there is some basis to the belief that self-awareness is not a fixed commodity, as its extent really depends on the persistence of our curious nature.

The reason though for that rather terse account, on the subject of our mental faculties, is because I have endeavored to employ the proposed notion of our mind in exploring the relationship between the actual directing and our spatial interpretation of any contorting we compel. For it is through our sense of self-awareness, reflecting our mind in action, that we are able to selectively filter any incoming sensory stimuli, from any one to all five senses. The discussion however will be confined primarily to our sense of touch since our ability to effectively control any contorting of our body is in part based on this rather complex set of sensory transducers, said to define just a single sense. Our sense of touch is then described here as complex because of not being constrained to a single intricate stimulus, such as with light or sound, as four different kinds of sensory information must be discerned, with each aspect having its own special type of sensory receptor. Although as perceived through an overall sensation of "feeling" the associated neural transducers can actually be divided into proximity sets, in effect defining an inner and an outer sense of touch. In school however, as denoted by the two distinct kinds of sensory receptors embedded within and below our skin, I only recall having to remember the specific attributes of our more tangibly accessible outer sense of touch. Since not just one type as a variety of structural configurations are actually employed, as neural transducers; thereby allowing for several different interpretations of the stimulus described here simply as pressure, usually from physical contact. Now the other distinct type of sensory receptor, whose nerve endings also permeate our dermis layer, is less involved because of having only two variations; with one kind that responds to an elevating in temperature and a complementary version, which only triggers when our skin is being cooled down. And so as defined by our perception of the transduced signals, from a multitude of pressure and thermal sensory receptors, our use of the word "feel" is attributed mainly to our outer sense of touch.

Seemingly then compared to our tactile sense the second set of sensory receptors, defining our inner sense of touch, are somehow perceived as being less noteworthy. The obvious reason of course, for this apparent oversight, is because the neural transducers that make-up our inner sense of touch are not superficially located near the surface of our skin but reside deep within our muscles and tendons. Probably more important though is the fact that, unlike with pressure or thermal sensory receptors, our inner sense of touch isn't viewed as being an independent indicator, since its presence is only really noted through the contracting of our skeletal musculature. And so as an integral part of our nervous system our inner sense of touch is considered mainly in the context of being a reactive feedback; denoting merely the return portion of an overall neural control loop, through which we direct any movement of our body. For any contorting we compel, through muscle tensing, is reflected through the electrochemical feedback from two distinct kinds of sensory receptors.

The first type of neural transducer, defining our inner sense of touch, is then nothing more than specially "wired" muscle tissue that through noting the difference in the resulting overlap, from the associated muscle group contracting, essentially conveys the degree of spatial displacement affected by some part of our body. And embedded in most of our tendons, connecting skeletal muscle to bone, is the other type of sensory receptor also defining our inner sense of touch. Here though a distortion gauge is the structure employed, as a neural transducer, to assess the amount of force generated by the attending muscle fibers contracting. And so through quantifying force and displacement, from a multitude of stretch and tension receptors, is what allows for our being cognizant of our body's spatial positioning, without any visual referencing from our eyes. Initially of course visual sensory feedback is probably crucial to developing a set degree of kinesthetic awareness, also known as our sense of proprioception. Whereby from years of simply improving on the incisiveness of our initiating gradually our cerebellum restructures itself to become so adept, at the spatial decoding of force and displacement feedback, we are able to least mimic any defined motion, even with our eyes closed.

Now just as we have two subtly distinct ways of consciously interpreting visual sensory information, through a "surveying" or a "scrutinizing" perspective, each hemispheric lobe of our cerebrum also has its own way of discerning sensory feedback from muscle activity. And so with our left cerebral cortex, designed for serial processing, our inner sense of touch would be closely correlated with the neural database of our cerebellum where, from relating to visual cues, stretch and tension feedback is initially encoded into defining our body's spatial positioning. This acute interface, between our cerebellum and the left hemispheric lobe of our cerebrum, is then the mechanism by which inner sensory feedback is more readily perceived in reference to how the efferent control signals should "feel", when performing a previously integrated motion sequence. Which is to say when engaged in any type of physical movement, initiated strictly by an already defined neural firing sequence, I envision our mindset as being characterized by a single left-brain metaphysical component, descriptively referred to as "active control".

But although oftentimes used in isolation active control is also an integral part of what constitutes a sensory mindset employing both hemispheric lobes of our cerebrum, in the discerning of inner sensory feedback. With just our right cerebral cortex however sensory information processing, from the stretch and tension receptors defining the muscles being used, is not directly correlated to spatial positioning, as with active control of our left cerebrum. Because with the concurrent analysis scheme of the right hemispheric lobe of our brain there is no acute referencing, for like our surveying view of the forest no single aspect is being scrutinized instead an overall assessing of relationships is being done. Therefore by defining, as related to inner sensory feedback, a "perceiving" rather than "controlling" nature to our mindset I refer to this particular right-brain metaphysical component as simply "passive sensing". And so by itself passive sensing would be employed as merely an intensity gauge, while at least moderately active, to determine how hard our muscles are working. In theory this assessing of physical effort is done through a summing or reducing of all inner sensory feedback into a singular sensation, commonly referred to as our perceived degree of exertion. Although as elaborated on in the next chapter this codifying into a singularity is presumed to be a generic form of sensory evaluation, applied not only to the electrochemical signals emanating from the sensory receptors of both our inner and outer (tactile) sense of touch but also our other four senses as well.

Additionally however to improve on our ability to precisely perform either a single motion or a whole series of exacting contortions as alluded to passive sensing is also used in conjunction with active control, the contrived metaphysical component of our left hemispheric lobe. Where through merely implementing a slower more methodical directing (of any attached appendage) we also tend to concurrently invoke an enhancing in the acuity of our spatial discerning, as a way to more readily assess the incisiveness of our initiating. And so as physiologically reflected through an increase in interfacing (between the two hemispheric lobes of our brain) the usual way of engaging, what I call a sensory mindset, is by just restraining the alacrity of our emulating to the slower pace of deliberate directing. Of course once we become relatively adept at replicating a particular motion it then becomes a more formidable task keeping passive sensing actively engaged, for any extended period of time. And so through the sheer number of contrived contortions employed is how the practice of Tai Chi is able to more readily maintain acute muscle control, as our perceptual sense of directing, even for relatively extended periods of time. Because with other exacting physical activities such as golf and tennis, due to their innate simplicity, it is only when initially emulating the various contortions employed, that we tend to consciously invoke an increase in the acuity of spatial discerning. The more enduring adaptation response however, from any periodic engaging of a sensory focus, being similar in that, from the accrued time maintaining acute muscle control, there is usually a related enhancing in the incisiveness of our initiating.

On the other hand because of the high level of resistance normally employed is one reason why the practice of overload conditioning is not exactly an ideal choice, from our engaging of a sensory focus, as a means of inducing a more enduring augmenting in our degree of kinesthetic awareness. For the problem being that, when maximizing impedance, our perceived degree of physical stress quickly reaches a point where, even though deliberately directing movement, our ability to maintain acute muscle control is severely curtailed. My rationale for this inability of ours to readily engage a sensory focus is then based on the notion that, when the intensity of stretch and tension feedback reaches a certain level, our inherent response is to just maintain active control. This restraining of our mental faculties is however merely a secondary effect from any physically demanding activity because, through the injury preventing mechanism commonly described as physical pain, our inner sense of touch is also employed to effectively limit the extent to which we are able to excel. Although through restricting our ability to persevere this incurred effect, from stretch and tension feedback, was probably what led to the premature passing of a number of our early ancestors, being primarily the prey and not the dominant predator that man is today. However since it allows for a certain increase in physical capacity, so as to better escape an impending threat, an ability to suppress our perception of force and displacement feedback was probably a trait readily acquired by our early descendants. I refer to that mindset, still employed today for excelling at physical extremes, as a high-intensity specific focus since there is also a related disposition of merely an explicit nature, which isn't usually directed at the suppressing of sensory feedback.

But as opposed to just my presumption presuming an evolutionary influence, on the possibility of a sensory suppressing mindset, there is also additional physiological evidence derived from a book that takes an in-depth look at the related neural circuitry of both our inner and outer sense of touch. That book *Job's Body: A handbook for Bodywork* is also where I got the idea that a limited intensifying of inner sensory feedback, while engaging a sensory focus, might be an effective way to circuitously improve on the incisiveness of our initiating, as related the physical contortions of our activity of choice. To briefly explain, as already mentioned, it is through our decoding of the conveyed inner sensory feedback, from the associated muscle spindles and Golgi tendon organs, that allows us to discern our body's spatial positioning, without the aid of our eyes. Implying that the high degree of control we normally exhibit, over any contorting of our body, is then the result of not just a single activation or efferent pathway. Because any movement we compel is usually achieved through the interaction between two sets of neural circuitry, with one path being efferent and the other afferent. Of the two though the descending motor pathways are generally the more acknowledged since they convey the efferent control signals that, through facilitating the contracting of our skeletal musculature, allow us to actually move. However because of being defined by both efferent and afferent neural pathways in effect that means our nervous system is functionally configured as a feedback-control loop. With the insinuation here being that, due to the operational scheme employed, rather than a single influence two sets of neural circuitry (both efferent and afferent) can actually be impacted on, from our engaging of a sensory focus.

Of course since our more common invoking of an increase in the acuity of our spatial discerning is to improve our ability to emulate an explicit motion that means any long-term impact, on our efferent neural pathways, would also be very specific. With our ascending sensory pathways however, from *any* maintaining of acute muscle control, our body's physiological response is relatively similar in being reflected through an overall induced lowering in impedance, to the conveyance of inner sensory feedback. This of course being in opposition to my earlier presumption that an integral function of our nervous system is in selectively filtering or essentially moderating the intensity of the electrochemical signals, emanating from the sensory receptors of our inner sense of touch. How then is it that we are able to impact on the prevailing impedance to the conveyance of inner sensory feedback, in both an affirmative and a contrary manner?

Well my understanding is that our ascending sensory pathways, which carry afferent sensory information to our brain, are overlaid with a series of descending neural pathways that are not efferent and so are not associated with eliciting the contracting of our skeletal musculature. Instead by synapsing to our ascending sensory pathways the interconnected descending neural pathways are employed, as a kind of gain control mechanism, for selectively filtering afferent sensory information from both our tactile and the sensory receptors of our inner sense of touch. And so the increase in the acuity of our spatial discerning, from engaging a sensory focus, is then essentially a result of our ascending neural circuits being directed, by our descending sensory pathways, to act as a kind of "facilitator" in the conveyance of force and displacement feedback. On the other hand, with a high-intensity specific focus, we are compelled into invoking such a degree of selective filtering, through our descending sensory pathways, as to partially constrain the relaying of the electrochemical signals from both our inner and outer sense of touch. And with the mind over matter demonstrations of extreme tolerance, from some type of physical abuse to our skin, being the more noteworthy example of developing an overly effective sensory suppressing mindset.

More commonly though, such as when I first started weightlifting, it is during intense physical activity that we consciously focus on the repressing of stretch and tension feedback. With the long-term impact, from periodically affecting the selective filtering of our inner sense of touch, being in part what allows for an even greater augmenting in our ability to persevere. And so if only partaking in some form of physical conditioning, with the goal of always striving to excel, then the effects of sensory moderating, from engaging a high-intensity specific focus, are seen as a positive attribute. Because if we also participate in an exacting physical activity, such as golf or tennis, then the end result, from routinely engaging in the suppressing of sensory feedback, is postulated as being more deleterious in nature. Since our enabling of a high-intensity specific focus, from even moderately intense resistance-conditioning, could possibly offset (at least to a degree) the incurred sensory enhancing benefit of decreased impedance usually acquired from a routine of reiterating with methodical precision, the integrated contortions of our exacting activity of choice.

But besides the deliberate practicing of our preferred activity my contention being that other techniques can likewise be employed which, albeit exhibiting a superficial variation in our disposition, achieve at least a comparable adaptation response in terms of the incurred diminishing in the prevailing impedance to the conveyance of inner sensory feedback. Primarily though I singled out the practice of Tai Chi which, due to the sheer number of contrived contortions employed, readily allowed for maintaining acute muscle control, even for extended periods of time. With dual sensory approach however, which is what this book elaborates on, rather than just another variation on either aforementioned explicit mindset, as a means of invoking an increase in the acuity of our spatial discerning, instead I have extended to employ a disposition of a more ambiguous nature. And so unlike with both methods considered earlier where, through emulating either a simple motion or a complex contortion, each one essentially relies on the eliciting attribute of incisiveness, to maintain acute muscle control. My approach to engaging a sensory focus is a bit more unconventional in really being just a concise overload conditioning routine.

Originally though the reason for my employing the four lifting motions, which constitute a dual sensory approach, was because of defining a fairly thorough exercise routine, for stressing the various musculature of my upper-body. Because with my decreed constraint, emphasizing equilateral utilization, each lifting motion is done in such a way that effectively engages both complementary sets of skeletal musculature, within our upper-arm and upper torso. Usually though with this particular setup, due to our inclination to focus on our extremities, we tend to consciously compel just the musculature of our upper-arm into being the prime mover. And so similar to the imposed mental constraint of every exercise of my upper-body strengthening routine, with a dual sensory approach, a part of our focus is also directed towards a more equitable engaging of the musculature of our upper-torso. However rather than just trying to compel a particular muscle group, into being the prime mover, a dual sensory mindset also calls for actually striving to improve on our perceiving of this subtle disparity, between the two ways of initiating the directing of our arms. Usually though from partaking in any type of physical activity, through a summing or reducing into a singular sensation, our discerning of inner sensory feedback is relegated to merely conveying an overall sense, as to how much effort we are exerting. Although due to the increased intensity of inner sensory feedback, from lifting weights, in effect that means the induced physical stress on our body's lever system is also what more acutely defines our spatial perception of our body's physical positioning. My contention however being that by just actively seeking a more perceptible sense for each manner of initiating, through our arms or from our shoulders, we are essentially eliciting an increase in the acuity of our spatial discerning, thus the basis to a dual sensory focus.

Now also related to this notion of there being a discernible difference, in primary upper-body limb control, I propose that the underlying reason the contortions employed are so difficult to master, in certain activities of skill, is because of our having two subtly distinct ways of implementing the flexing of either arm. Where with our inherent inclination, to center our focus point of control on our hand or wrist, it is almost impossible to generate, with any consistency, the exacting power needed to excel in any number of exacting physical activities, not just golf and tennis. For achieving such rapid arm movement, with at least a fair degree of accuracy, requires having developed a sense of control that, as best I can explain, is not maintained at just a singular position. As years of working on my tennis game have led to employing what I perceive as a "moving apex of manipulation" which only becomes fixed, on my wrist or hand, just before contacting the ball. Although it was only after I started diligently practicing with deliberate precision, the full swing motion of both my backhand and forehand, that I was ultimately able to really develop a sense for a shifting point of control. Since the more enduring effect, from engaging in a routine of meticulously reiterating either tennis stroke, was to allow for a shifting in my spatial perception, from being constrained to a fixed point, to encompassing a sense of the entire motion. All of which of course resulted in the rather abrupt increase in both the accuracy and potency of my tennis strokes.

And so extending on this concept of a disparity in primary upper-body limb control I propose that our maintaining of acute shoulder control, to consciously isolate a particular muscle group, is very similar (in terms of movement origin) to what is normally employed when reiterating, with deliberate precision, the full swing motion of either a backhand or forehand stroke. Implying that it is only in pace of movement where the difference lies in our sense of directing, between precision power (in sports) and exacting shoulder control (when lifting weights). Briefly detailing this notion, on the importance of acquiring a sense of acute upper-torso control, is then rather self-explanatory in regards to it denoting, with a dual sensory focus, the importance of the decreed mental constraint on active control, in the compelling of any flexing of either arm.

A dual sensory approach, as embodied in a concise four-exercise lifting routine, is then my proposal of a remedy for those who engage in some sort of exacting physical activity but can never seem to practice enough to maintain, on a consistent basis, a sense of acute shoulder control. Which is to say this mental technique really developed out of my own frustration, for over fifteen years, with the game of tennis. However after several weeks of following the guidelines described herein a lot of that aggravation finally came to an end. Since the more enduring effect of my enhanced sense of proprioception, from engaging a dual sensory focus, was in seemingly exaggerating my perception of any mistakes I made while playing tennis. Although as reflected through an augmenting in the consistency of my tennis strokes a keener sense of what occasionally went wrong actually translated into a better feel, for how to avoid making unforced errors. Over time however it also became apparent that the increase in the acuity of my spatial discerning was not the only benefit to be had, from employing a dual sensory approach. Because by affecting the palpability of our sense of touch, which essentially establishes the basis to our physical presence, it would seem to follow that there would also be some sort of corresponding impact related to our mental psyche. Discussion on that topic however relating to the more abstract mental accommodations incurred, from employing a dual sensory approach, I have reserved for the final chapter.

The reason though for such a detailed introduction, briefly discussing all the insights and presumptions on which a dual sensory approach is based, is of course because of possibly being dismissed as just another lifting routine. For where the sensory enhancing benefits lie, from the lifting motions employed, is through our effective use of an elusive concept referred to simply as passive sensing. But rather than go into lengthy discourse explaining just exactly how it could all possibly work the goal here (with this book) is merely to further develop my functional denoting of our brain/mind, as based on the bilateral processing of sensory information. Therefore my writing will continue to be concise, which may oversimplify things somewhat, but that should allow for a more effective incorporating of the sensory enhancing technique elaborated on over the course of next two chapters and so not limiting one to just the more routine augmenting in function, usually acquired from the practice of resistance conditioning.

Chapter 1

Passive Sensing

Initially then passive sensing will be considered by itself in a singular or isolated context and so theoretically in terms of sensory information processing by just the right hemispheric lobe of our bilateral brain. Because when interfacing with active control of our left cerebral cortex is at a minimum then, through a summing or reducing of stretch and tension feedback into a singular sensation, passive sensing is constrained to being employed as merely a gauge of physical exertion. Where in the extreme, in terms of the transduced sensory stimuli from both our inner and outer sense of touch, this codifying into a singularity is tangibly described as simply physical pain. At lesser degrees of incurred duress however the term "intense" is oftentimes used not only as a means of defining our degree of physical effort but also as a descriptive reference, for quantifying sensory feedback from our other four senses. In effect alluding to passive sensing being employed as an intensity gauge not only for our sense of touch but also our sense of hearing, smell, taste and sight. So for example, with audio processing, passive sensing would be directed at just assessing how loud a particular sound, irrespective of its origin. As for both taste and smell the measure of intensity, by passive sensing, would be through judging strictly chemical concentration, regardless of composition. And as for visual stimuli, to define intensity, passive sensing would simply gauge the radiance of the light striking the cones and rods, covering the back of our eyes. But as merely an appraiser of physical effort what are the external factors, from engaging in any type of physical activity, that actually have an impact on passive sensing, in regards to establishing our perceived degree of effort or intensity?

Well with simple repetitious motion as the basis to almost every form of fitness conditioning, from augmenting strength to improving on our stamina, that defines rate of movement and resistance to motion as the two essential attributes, affecting our sense of the incurred physical stress. If however the primary consideration being developing strength of these two attributes, whose combined impact determines our perceived degree of intensity, resistance to motion is usually the more predominant. Because with an aerobic exercise impedance to motion must be kept at such a low level that if invariable the prevailing attribute, defining our sense of how much physical effort we are exerting, shifts to being just rate of movement. Of course with many types of aerobic exercise machines, along with how fast we move our arms and legs, the slight altering of resistance to motion is also oftentimes employed, as an additional way to impact on the degree of physical effort required. If however, as a rather extreme example, impedance to motion were to steadily increase then, to sustain movement, the number of enabled muscle fibers would reach a point where a once predominately aerobic exercise now becomes an activity more anaerobic in nature. With that transition, from aerobic to predominately anaerobic, being of course perceived as simply an augmenting in the degree of physical effort required. Although physiologically this transition in cellular respiration is in fact denoted through increasingly employing what are called "fast" twitch muscle fibers, in lieu of our other type of skeletal musculature known as "slow" twitch. This distinction between developing strength and stamina is then reflected not only through a difference in the actual cellular energy-releasing process being employed, either "aerobic" or "anaerobic", as each applied term is also associated with the difference between which type of muscle fiber is primarily engaged during each type of activity.

So what allows us to endure, under physically demanding workloads, is essentially an ability to continue initiating muscle contractions, even though oxygen is not readily available as an energizing force. And although extreme physical exertion can only be sustained for brief periods of time with a short rest, if not too overcome by fatigue, we are able to repeat an intense physical activity for several sets (if we happen to be weightlifting) or intervals (if partaking in speed training). Therefore in chapter four "Aerobic Conditioning" the localized effects, from engaging in some form of physical activity, are further considered from the perspective of cellular respiration and not the three related factors that actually define what benefits will be incurred, if any, from following a prescribed exercise routine.

Now since it initially establishes where the impact will be primarily felt, in terms of conveying some kind of adaptation response, that makes our perceived degree of physical exertion the first attribute to be considered, with regards to any type of fitness conditioning program. Because if the workload of an exercise is very demanding, either in terms of pace or resistance, then although both types of musculature may be engaged it is virtually impossible to maintain the activity long enough, therefore limiting any physiological response to affecting mainly fast-twitch muscle fibers. If however impedance to motion is relatively low and our pace of movement not too expeditious then the second factor duration comes into play, as now both ways of harnessing cellular energy (through either aerobic or anaerobic means) can be significantly enhanced. Because if an activity of sufficient intensity is maintained for a long enough period of time then not only are all the muscle fibers engaged affected, both fast-twitch and slow-twitch, as a slew of other adaptations may also be incurred. Usually though, as brought on by any type of aerobic activity, the more noted physiological response being the impact on the function of our heart and lungs.

This differential though, between the amount of time needed to develop either strength or stamina, is enough to make for two different ways of denoting the activity period for either type of exercise. Where with almost every kind of resistance conditioning routine, isometric being the exception, duration can be expressed through simply counting the number of repetitions completed, as the actual time spent lifting is usually no more than a minute or two. On the other hand, with an aerobic activity, the number of recurring motions that must be performed is so great as to make elapsed time a better method of gauging duration, rather than counting repetitions. Time also allows for, in relation to a set interval, readily defining an actual pace; thereby numerically quantifying the variable of intensity, whereas merely knowing the number of steps to cover a certain distance says nothing about the degree of effort required.

The third factor, affecting the adaptation response of our body, is the variable of frequency and it is actually used in two different instances, depending on the time frame employed. Initially then, over the course of a single workout, frequency is used to denote the number of times a particular activity is to be performed, as stipulated by the prescribed exercise routine. And so with an overload conditioning program frequency would simply define the set count for each exercise of a set routine. Now intriguing though it may be there is just no way of designating a single repetition series as having preeminence over all others, since the ideal number of times to perform an exercise is really determined by the specifics of one's goal. A lifting sequence of just three sets, with each one consisting of between eight to twelve repetitions, is however what is considered optimal for the general conditioning of all related sets of skeletal musculature, employed in initiating any movement of either our arms or legs.

Additionally of course, in terms of speed conditioning or interval training, frequency is also used to denote the number of times a set distance is to be traversed, through some type of physical locomotion. With a strictly aerobic conditioning program however frequency is essentially reduced to one, since the primary consideration being merely the total time spent active. Although the set interval of activity defined as optimal, in terms of the adaptation response it induces, can actually vary from ten to thirty minutes, depending on our perceived degree of exertion. And so what in fact denotes the impact of the physical stress incurred, from engaging in some form of aerobic conditioning, is then not just duration or how long we remain physically active but also intensity, as reflected through our perceived degree of exertion. With the basis to these conclusions, about the physiological adaptations brought on by aerobic exercise, being further discussed in chapter three "The Program" where the concept of optimal fitness, in regards to developing either strength or stamina, is considered in the context of diminishing returns.

Finally then, over the long-term, frequency is used to denote (usually over the set interval of a week) the number of workouts required for simply sustaining or significantly improving upon a certain aspect of fitness, in this case either strength or stamina. And so to enhance our aerobic capacity, as defined through oxygen uptake, would mean engaging in anywhere from three workouts over a seven-day period to exercising every day of the week, depending on the relative intensity and duration of each activity. To merely retain muscle tone however, through some form of resistance conditioning, would entail just one workout a week, which thoroughly engages all applicable sets of skeletal musculature. Of course to more readily induce the desired physiological response of increasing size and strength would require partaking in at least two lifting sessions a week; with some programs allowing just a forty-eight hour respite for the various sets of skeletal musculature, employed by a defined routine. Now in spite of my fitness-related goal being simply the prevention of muscle atrophy I actually prefer working out twice a week, as I feel the increased frequency is more optimal for maintaining and even possibly improving on my degree of kinesthetic awareness.

In summary as reflected physiologically through either the incurred increase in oxygen uptake or decrease, in the rhythmic contractions of our heart, to extend on our ability to endure would require partaking in at least ten minutes of continuous activity, depending on our perceived degree of exertion. And so through merely pace of movement and/or by also varying resistance to motion, with almost every aerobic activity, at least one of two means can be employed, to impact on the physiological adaptation response incurred by our body. In contrast strength is usually gained by exercising for about a minute or two and most of the time the only mechanism used, to affect our sense of the incurred physical stress, is through altering impedance to motion. Because rather than lifting more or less weight, to impact on the degree of effort required, the varying of pace is not oftentimes employed, except by those in the more advanced stages of bodybuilding. The reason though as I see it, why altering the tempo of lifting is not generally considered an option, is because of what happens to our sense of the incurred physical stress, when the level of impedance defines a primarily muscle strengthening exercise.

Because rather than a decrease in exertion, which comes from slowing down a repetitious activity of minimal limb impedance, at some point as resistance is increased an inverse effect is incurred where, instead of a diminishing, deliberate movement tends to affect an escalation in the amount physical effort required. With this counterintuitive consequence, affecting our perception of how much effort we are exerting, being of course reflected through our tendency to lift moderate to heavy objects rather quickly instead of slowly, which would seem to require less effort. Therefore in chapter three "The Program" there is a brief detailing on the actual cause of this inverse effect of increasing our sense of the incurred physical stress, whenever deliberately lifting anything of significant impedance.

In this chapter however while engaged in some sort of physical activity, although a number of potential variations in our disposition will be elaborated on, only one example will make use of the aforementioned inverse effect of increased resistance. And so instead of any of the resistance-based conditioning exercises from the as yet to be discussed dual sensory lifting program, through the everyday activity of placing one foot in front of the other, mainly a variation in pace of movement will be employed, to distinguish between three types of mental focus. Coincidentally there are also three reasons for choosing walking; the first one being that, as a thoroughly integrated neural firing sequence, for most of us the degree of conscious oversight required is at a minimum, entailing just active control. Secondly even for a marginally fit person casually placing one foot in front of the other is usually not that strenuous; thereby allowing for a more effortless extending of our use of passive sensing, beyond merely assessing effort. Finally the ease of increasing the degree of effort required, through simply moving faster, allows for readily discerning the perceptual difference between what I see as the two extremes in our disposition, defining the extent over which we actively engage our cerebellum. Where at the low end of the intensity spectrum our mindset of choice being usually a general focus of a more distracted nature. If however the effort required becomes more physically demanding, through an increase in either pace of movement or resistance to motion, we would be compelled (at some point) to engage a high-intensity specific focus, as a way of somewhat easing our mental duress. Of course the actual transition marking this distinction, between a general mindset and high-intensity specific focus, is to a large degree under our conscious control. After a certain point however switching to a sensory moderating mindset simply becomes an instinctive response. And so through first employing just pace of movement, from running in this case, the following example is meant to illustrate that what ultimately establishes our sense of the incurred physical stress is actually the interaction between both genetics and conditioning, although oftentimes the latter is initially a significant factor.

Initially then my attributes of an average runner will be compared with a hypothetical person I call "Swifty", named so because of being endowed with the potential to be a world-class athlete. Now if Swifty never develops his inherent advantage, through training on a regular basis, then running would always be a very physically demanding activity after just a short period of time, even at my relatively slow pace. Although rather than from just stretch and tension feedback, from the skeletal musculature employed, the underlying sense for Swifty's perception of physical effort is increasingly based on the accumulation of lactic acid that, due to a lack of conditioning, isn't readily removed. For any progressive lowering in the pH level of the affected intracellular solution tends to invoke, from any further contracting by the associated skeletal musculature, a related intensifying in our perception of physical pain; consequently forcing Swifty to slow down if not completely stop. Should Swifty however develop his innate talent, through some sort of aerobic activity, then a relatively moderate pace for him would probably be very physically demanding for me. Although any athlete without the associated genetic advantage would struggle to keep pace with one so gifted, not just me. And so based on not just a set level of aerobic fitness our ability to excel is also defined by any number of inherent constraints on design which are oftentimes a compensation that allows for an enhancing in our performance, at other extreme of the fitness spectrum.

Once again however, as reflected in the actual lifting that I do, it would appear that I am also not especially gifted, if instead of stamina a comparison of strength had been done. As probably quite a few individuals could be found who have never endeavored to partake in bodybuilding but are still able to lift more than I ever could, regardless of how much I train. For although an initial lack of fitness always tends to deleteriously impact on our ability to contend, in terms of strength however oftentimes it is still not enough to offset an inherent advantage. But because greater strength is usually associated with having more physical mass that means this aspect of genetics can be and actually is selectively applied in the competitive arena, through some sports having different weight classes. In other sporting events though there is no discrimination based on weight, implying that having a size advantage over one's opponent does not necessarily translate into a competitive edge or so they say.

But enough conjecture on the advantage of size as it is time to define (as related to almost any kind of physical activity) not only each outlying disposition, over the extent that we actively enable our cerebellum, but also an invoking of a more intermediary nature. And so first up a general focus, the mindset most commonly employed during all low to moderate levels of physical exertion. Next a sensory focus, which of course reflects our maintaining of acute muscle control. And finally a high-intensity specific focus; which was defined as the mindset we inherently tend to invoke, as our sense of the incurred workload becomes increasingly more demanding.

Now by simply walking on a strip of level ground where resistance to motion is rather nominal and one's pace not so fast, as to be overly strenuous after only a few minutes, is an easy way of getting a sense of what I call a general mindset. If however, from merely meandering, the effort involved starts to be perceived as very physically demanding, if not curtailed, our general focus would be compelled into becoming a sensory moderating mindset, as a way of alleviating the incurred increase in sensory discomfort. Should that occur, where walking for just a short distance turns into an arduous task, one might consider seeing a doctor about getting a physical checkup. Of course if there are any reservations about one's physical ability, before engaging in any kind of fitness conditioning regimen, reliable medical advice should initially be sought out.

Now if actually partaking in the ongoing inquiry the discerning of a general focus would have been denoted by an invoked division that allows us to engage in other mental diversions; while still successfully performing any seemingly simple repetitive motion, as for example walking. Because while the act of placing one foot in front of the other is by no means simple normally however, even at an early age, this rather complex maneuver of controlled falling is already a thoroughly integrated neural firing sequence. And so since it allows for the vagrancy of mind that some employ for self-reflection, while other seek distractions of a more appreciable nature, a general focus is functionally envisioned as being of a bilateral disposition.

The next phase of this demonstration then involves redirecting, into a sensory mindset, the available mental faculties of a general focus. And an easy way of doing that (of invoking a temporary increase in the acuity of our spatial discerning) is by extending from just walking to concentrating on making one's footfalls as light as possible, as if trying to sneak up on someone. Where in effect the mental diversions associated with a general focus are displaced, through our effort to improve on the incisiveness of our initiating. Which shows just how easy it is to engage a sensory mindset of maintaining acute muscle control, even though the complexity of the contortion involved being rather nominal.

But although readily enabled, through merely initiating a more meticulous directing of any compelled movement of our body, the problem is keeping passive sensing actively involved, as one may start to notice how much mental energy is really takes to consciously control one's footfalls. And so since simply placing one foot in front of the other doesn't normally necessitate our invoking of an augmenting in the acuity of our spatial discerning most of us would probably, in short order, go back to walking normally. Of course if we wanted to become more adept at performing a series of elaborate motions, such as learning Tai Chi, then it becomes more of a necessity, rather than an indulgence, to compel an increase in the incisiveness of our initiating.

Now one possible reason for our actually having to engage a sensory focus is because of the relatively nominal level of inner sensory feedback, which usually defines our maintaining of acute muscle control. And so to get a better "feel" for the associated stretch and tension transducers, related to the specific sets of skeletal musculature for compelling locomotion, stop walking and instead start doing a deep-knee bend. Because after squatting down, as reflected through an augmenting in the intensity of inner sensory feedback, the generalized sense of an increase in our perception of the incurred physical stress is also what acutely defines which leg and lower-back muscles are predominately being employed, when trying to straighten up. The reason though for this escalating in the contractile force needed, when extending from the deep-knee bend position, is because the structural design of both our knee and elbow joints is such that leverage distance, from the pivot point of the articulation being employed, actually changes with the flexing of either our arms or legs. And so through altering the mechanical advantage of the articulation in question the amount of applied force needed to lift a set weight will increase or decrease, with the changing angle of the joint or joints involved. This shifting in leverage distance, through the flexing of either our arms or legs, is then perceived as an augmenting or diminishing in our sense of strength where, at the extremes of almost fully extended or bent at an acute angle, either the function of pushing is regarded as being at its "strongest" and pulling at its "weakest" or vice versa. Specifically though, with either arm, this varying in the contractile force needed actually translates into our biceps, used for pulling, being perceived as most suspect when either elbow joint is almost fully extended and most secure, at the other extreme, when retracted at an angle of forty-five degrees or less. In contrast our triceps, employed for pushing, are sensed just the opposite way in being perceived as "strongest" when either arm is almost straight and "weakest" when either elbow joint is bent at an acute angle. Which is of course similar to how we sense our quadriceps, as can be readily discerned from actually doing a deep-knee bend.

Now the reason we are able to consciously register the fact that more muscle fibers are being employed, from doing a deep-knee bend, is of course because of the increase in both the number of stretch receptors concurrently active and in the firing rate of the associated tension transducers, already under stress. The end result however from all that heightened activity, by the sensory receptors of our inner sense of touch, is usually to simply invoke a relative sense of how much effort we are exerting. Although after a certain increase in incurred physical stress, from any arduous activity, our perceived degree of effort becomes so intense as to compel our neural processing system into suppressing inner sensory feedback, as a way to alleviate the incurred increase in sensory discomfort. Oftentimes though the actual means we tend to employ, as a way of easing our mental duress, being our conscious invoking of a more methodical breathing rhythm. And so as a way of allowing one to further excel, at some sort of physical activity, a high-intensity specific focus is in fact defined by an even more distinct bilateral mindset, than a general focus.

Finally then, for the last part of this demonstration, rather than an augmenting in resistance to motion, as the prevailing attribute, instead increased pace of movement will be employed, as the primary means of invoking a sensory moderating mindset. Because by just walking faster or actually running we inevitably get to a point where along with our breathing and heart rate being significantly accelerated, our ability to endure also starts to be adversely affected. However through engaging, what I refer to as a high-intensity specific focus, we are oftentimes able to persevere beyond the seemingly imposed limit on our physically excel.

Now if the possibility exists for inherently having an enhanced ability to affect the conveyance of the electrochemical signals defining our inner sense of touch, by extrapolating on a bell curve, it would only be conferred on about ten percent of the population. However having never really been exemplary, in any form of fitness conditioning I was to engage in, to the best of my knowledge any advantage incurred, from an augmenting in my ability at sensory suppressing, was probably not bestowed upon me. And at the other extreme, as defined by the consistency of my tennis game, the benefit from any possible sensory enhancing attribute had been nominal at best, until of course I started employing a dual sensory approach. For then in a relatively short period of time, from engaging a dual sensory focus, I was able to induce a more enduring increase in the acuity of my spatial discerning, even though when running I still defaulted to a sensory suppressing mindset. Because although our perception of intensity may be somewhat similar, in being sensed as physical pain, there is an underlying difference between sensory feedback based primarily on rate of movement versus resistance to motion. Leading to the contention that with certain types of physical conditioning, from our engaging of a sensory suppressing mindset, there is a lower probability of deleteriously impacting on the incisiveness of our initiating, as related to our exacting activity of choice. Specifically though with any exercise where intensity is varied mainly though pace, with only slight changes in a rather nominal resistance to motion.

But while invoking no more than a moderate degree of perceived intensity, from any kind of physical effort, despite the fact that engaging in either disposition is still relatively easy, versus sensory enhancing, our inherent tendency is towards the suppressing of inner sensory feedback. And although not really noted by runners in general, on the other hand, bodybuilders will oftentimes refer to the result, from periodically engaging in sensory moderating, as going "stale" from being so conditioned by a set routine that any tingling sensation, the exercises once possibly evoked, is no longer felt. I however through employing a completely different mindset have never perceived any type of staleness, as I have almost always been able to elicit at least a mild tingling sensation even after ten years of partaking in the same concise lifting routine.

That concludes my presentation for describing, as applied to really any physical activity, the difference in disposition between an easygoing and a Type-A personality. More importantly though, sandwiched between a casual and a more competitive approach, I defined a specific sensory focus where the more diverse utilization of a general mindset was effectively channeled into maintaining acute muscle control. In the next chapter however the engaging of a dual (or differentiating) sensory focus is considered because, at increased levels of physical exertion, a more ambiguous mindset is less inclined to affect a suppressing of inner sensory feedback, compared to a singular disposition.

Chapter 2

Acute Muscle Control

In the final part of the preceding chapter then, from the contrived exercise on perceptual discerning, I tried to establish a sense for each subtly distinct disposition where we actively interface with the actual initiating intermediary of our brain, which in fact coordinates the contracting of our skeletal musculature. And so over the extent that we actively employ our cerebellum, the alluded to intermediary, my original intent was to just compare the two extremes in our demeanor. Because at each outlying disposition, defined as either a general mindset or high-intensity specific focus, passive sensing is constrained to being employed as merely an intensity gauge, for conveying an overall sense of how much effort we are exerting. With the second mindset actually discussed however (between the two extremes) passive sensing was extended to encompass a more thorough discerning, beyond simply assessing effort. Where through merely compelling a more deliberate directing (of how our footfalls make contact with the ground) we also tend to concurrently induce an interim increase in the acuity of our spatial discerning, which at times can actually make maintaining our balance more difficult. Although our invoking of this enhancing in the incisiveness of our initiating is usually an indicator that on some level, not always just consciously, we feel that our replicating of a particular motion could be more exacting.

Our engaging of a sensory focus, to maintain acute muscle control, is then not just for extending an immediate augmenting in the precision of our emulating of an exacting physical contortion. Since the more enduring benefit, from invoking an interim increase in the acuity of our spatial discerning, is usually to improve on our long-term ability to precisely replicate the particular motion, which was subject to acute muscle control. Although ordinarily the only time we tend to consciously engage an explicit sensory mindset, in an effort to improve on the incisiveness of our initiating, is when initially implementing the optimal neural firing sequence defining a particular motion. Of course oftentimes later on, usually after having erred once or twice, we are once again compelled into maintaining acute muscle control, in an effort to improve on our emulating of a particular motion. Because even though our nervous system can be conditioned into being a very exacting mechanism, to precisely control any contorting of our body, for the most part we humans are not very precise, possibly due in part to our extended range of motion. For even after neural integration, through a program of reiteration, duplicating a seemingly simple motion sequence, such as a golf or tennis stroke, with the precision that it was previously performed, while not impossible, is extremely difficult given a small margin of error. Through additional practice however of any exacting motion sequence an even greater reduction in our overall degree of deviation can usually be achieved, although the complexity involved in implementing any deliberate contorting of our body keeps our response from ever being purely mechanical.

Unlike however our maintaining of acute muscle control for improving on the incisiveness of our initiating, the emphasis of a dual sensory focus is not primarily on the motion being performed. Instead our mindset is directed at just striving to improve on our perceiving of this subtle disparity in our focus point of manipulation, as sensed from either our hands or invoked through our shoulders. With the idea being that we are essentially compelling an increase in the acuity of our spatial discerning by just trying to get a better feel for this difference in our sense of directing, as perceived from either our hands or invoked through our shoulders. And at levels of resistance considered moderately intense my contention being that rather than a specific focus, with its tendency towards sensory moderating, a more effective way of maintaining acute muscle control is through engaging a dual sensory mindset. But although more tolerant to the persuasive influence of physical stress, in ease of sensing, a dual sensory focus is really restricted to a rather limited number of motions encompassed mainly, in terms of muscle usage, by the four lifting exercises elaborated on in the next chapter.

At exertion levels of merely limb resistance then, as exemplified by the intricate articulations employed by Tai Chi, acute muscle control is usually sustained through engaging an explicit sensory focus. Although the ease at which an increase in the acuity of our spatial discerning could be invoked was actually demonstrated, in the last chapter, by merely initiating a more deliberate compelling of our basic mode of locomotion. Of course unlike with Tai Chi and its convoluted contortions walking is a fairly integrated motion sequence and so our engaging of a sensory mindset is really just to compel an increase in the acuity of our spatial discerning, rather than actually trying to improve on the incisiveness of our initiating. My contention though being that the same elevating in our degree of kinesthetic awareness can in fact be invoked through either subtly distinct disposition, with an inclination towards merely sensing or the actual directing of any contorting of our body.

But besides providing initial force and displacement information to our cerebellum, the conveyance of which every sensory focus tries to improve upon, inner sensory feedback also functions as a safety mechanism that, in the extreme, is employed to actually limit the extent to which we are able to physically excel. Of some consequence then, especially if we compete in some type of physical activity, this somewhat debilitating effect of our inner sense of touch was of course depicted as a fatal detriment to early man, who was still an easy prey to a number of predators. However since it allows for an interim increase in physical capacity, so as to better escape an impending danger, the more adaptive of our descendants were probably the first to actually employ, what I call as a sensory moderating mindset. And so through exploiting an inherent survival mechanism of our early ancestors is how we today are able to persevere, beyond the prevailing threshold normally imposed on us by the pain of extreme physical exertion. That then being my simple evolutionary account of what allows us to, in response to any significant increase in our incurred workload, maintain our degree of effort through engaging a high-intensity specific focus.

And so compared to a specific mindset, with its tendency towards the suppressing of sensory feedback, the advantage of a dual sensory focus then being that even under a fair amount mental duress, as brought on by resistance to motion, keeping this rather ambiguous disposition actively enabled is relatively easy, if distractions are not taken into account. Whereby from just trying to elicit a keener sense for each manner of compelling the directing of either arm, with an inclination towards our hands or through our shoulders, our mindset isn't relegated to the singularity of a specific focus, to still actively maintain acute muscle control. And so to get a better feel for this disparity the following discussion leads up to describing each subtly distinct way of implementing the flexing of either arm; first with our focus point of control as perceived from our hands and then with a sense of initiating, as invoked through our shoulders.

Initially then, in terms of physiology, movement of either arm is of course not limited to being controlled by just the skeletal musculature located within each upper-arm. For almost any varying of spatial positioning is additionally augmented by actively engaging, at least through structural support, the skeletal muscle groups contained within our upper-torso. Usually though since our focus point of control is directed at our hands it is the musculature of our upper-arm, our biceps and triceps, that are compelled into doing most of the work, with any flexing of either arm. However through simply redirecting our mental focus, to a sense of initiating through our shoulders, that should allow for a more equitable engaging of each complementary set of skeletal musculature, within our upper-arm and upper-torso. Although when using a barbell, through a simple shift in physical placement, it is also possible to effectively restrict our range of motion to target just one particular muscle group, within our upper-arm or upper-torso, irrespective of our invoked disposition. The last part of this chapter then initially elaborates on the two ways of lifting a barbell that although employing the same basic flexing motion, depending on a slight setup adjustment, a different set of skeletal musculature (within our upper-arm or upper-torso) is directed into being the prime mover.

But based on this disparity in our conscious initiating, as sensed from our hands or invoked through our shoulders, my denoting of a distinction originally evolved out of a division where the only premise for defining a difference was in either being a pushing out or pulling in motion. Because through either a normal or converse implementation of our body's lever system of muscles, bones, ligaments and tendons almost any lifting exercise can be reduced to merely a sense of extending or retracting. Of course this rather rudimentary approach to differentiating different lifting motions was not of my doing as it was already discussed in *The 'Sports Illustrated' Book On Weightlifting*, where I first read about it.

Normal lifting, in one sense, then entails our system of bone levers being controlled by a complementary tandem of skeletal musculature that, through contracting, compels the implement of impedance (we happen to holding) to be brought closer to us. The same holds true for the converse implementation where we do the moving, to try and pull ourselves up, as what we are grasping usually remains fixed. With the other rudimentary function however, where force must be exerted in the extending of our arms, only the same bones and ligaments of our lever system are primarily engaged, when performing either a normal or a converse lifting activity. Because a separate complementary tandem of skeletal musculature and attending tendons are employed, within our upper-arm and upper-torso, when we partake in any type of physical effort where the intent is to increase our degree of detachment from the implement of impedance we happen to be holding. And although usually of no concern when our primary goal, from engaging in some form of resistance conditioning, is to simply augment the amount of weight we are able to lift. On the other hand, as a way of increasing muscle definition, the more exacting discipline of bodybuilding does extend to employing specific exercises designed explicitly for isolating (of an affected tandem) just one particular muscle group, either within our upper-arm or upper-torso.

Now as opposed to a single set the advantage of a functional tandem (of comparably employed musculature) is of course in the extended range of motion it allows for, compared to contorting through just a single articulation. Also due to the complementary nature of the interaction between the various sets of skeletal musculature, within our upper-arm and upper-torso, oftentimes that means there is at least a partial summing of the contractile force generated by each affected muscle group. Although due to our inherent tendency to focus on our extremities more often than not it is just the musculature of our upper-arm, either our biceps or triceps, that are directed into being the prime mover. However since it does allow for increasing the total contractile force possible, whenever lifting anything relatively heavy, we are oftentimes compelled into invoking a more equitable engaging of both affected sets of skeletal musculature, within our upper-arm and upper-torso. And so through an understanding of each manner of deliberately directing either arm, with a dual sensory approach, the idea is to just try and get a better sense for this disparity in our sense of control. Now to consider our conscious compelling of either arm; first with our focus point of control as centered on our hand and then with a perception of initiating, as invoked through our shoulder.

Each arm of course, on either side of our body, is structurally quite complex although most of the defined skeletal musculature lies below our elbow for controlling our thumb and four fingers, usually on each hand. And so in regards to gross manipulation the only muscles groups of concern are the two situated above either elbow joint; namely our biceps, used for retracting, and our triceps, employed whenever force is needed in the extending of either arm. As directed primarily by our triceps then an acute sense of reaching out would be perceived as simply a straightening of the three skeletal structures (two in our forearm and one in our upper-arm) on either side of each elbow joint. On the other hand the withdrawing of either arm, by just our biceps, would invoke just the opposite sensation of being perceived as merely a sense of bending at the elbow. But although having seemingly defined our sense of initiating as originating from either elbow joint in both instances however, when movement is compelled by primarily the musculature of our upper-arm, our center of attention is actually directed at the distal end of our forearm. In effect our perception of manipulation is spatially sensed, from the perspective of our hands, more in terms of shifting from point A to point B (as for example grasping a cup and moving it towards our mouth) and so not just in terms of how our elbows flex. "Point-to-point" then being a more definitive way of describing our sense of directing, versus simply extending or retracting, since the control of either arm is almost always augmented, at least through structural support, by the musculature of our upper-torso.

Our upper-body of course, even without its attending appendages, also consists of a significant number of muscles groups although what will be considered here are just the three predominant sets of skeletal musculature, which primarily control the spatial positioning of each upper-arm. Initially then a single large back muscle, the latissmus dorsi, is what compels any retracting of our arms by just our upper-torso. In contrast two relatively smaller muscle groups, the pectorals and deltoids, are each employed either separately or in conjunction, whenever force is needed in the extending of either upper-arm. Although to actually affect any movement the various muscles groups, contained within our upper-torso, must transfer the force of contracting through a complex structure known mechanically as a ball-and-socket joint. And from our engaging of the various sets of skeletal musculature, which affect movement through either shoulder joint, it is of course fairly obvious that a much greater range of motion is allowed for, compared to the mere reaching and recanting by which either elbow joint is constrained. This increased freedom of movement, projected through our humerus bone, is then what led to the discerning of what can be called "defining angles" where just one particular upper-body muscle group is predominately employed, while other similar function musculature offers only nominal support. And so the basis to performing, at both the overhead and over-chest position, the same basic motion of pushing out, versus pulling in, is because the first locale (overhead) defines the angle for isolating our deltoids, while at the second position (over our chest) it is our pectoral muscles that are primarily engaged.

But although a common practice in bodybuilding this physical restricting of our utilization, to just a specific set of skeletal musculature, is of course contrary to what is employed with a dual sensory approach. Because rather than our innate way of directing either arm the only adjustment with a dual sensory approach being a mental one in the shifting of our internal center of attention up to each endpoint of control, which extends from either shoulder. Ultimately though what we are essentially doing, when consciously directing either arm through primarily the musculature constrained within our upper-body, is invoking a more equitable sense for all muscle groups actively involved, in both our upper-torso *and* upper-arm. Also when our sense of movement is compelled, through primarily our upper-torso, our range of motion is extended to encompass the more complex configuration of a three-dimensional cone, compared to the mere varying of a two-dimensional angle from any flexing by either elbow joint. Which is to say what actually defines the basis to the versatility of movement, exhibited by both our arms and legs, is the interaction between both flexing and gyrating. However by focusing on just the rotary component, through our shoulders, that should invoke an awareness of any wrist or elbow bending which is more passive in nature, with any physical adjustments now being made without any conscious oversight.

But although denoting our extended range of motion as encompassing a three-dimensional cone, with most resistance-conditioning exercises, movement is generally confined to a single plane, thereby relegating our sense of movement to a perception of "arc tracing". My analogy, depicting our sense of shoulder control, then being a reference to the workings of a mechanical compass where one leg is fixed consequently all movement of the free leg extends from a single point, descriptively the clamp on top but in actuality our shoulder joint. And so although defined at its base by a circle, with most forms of resistance conditioning, the full rotary motion of our humerus bone is constrained to encompassing merely a single arc where oftentimes extending increases its size, while recanting affects a decrease. This designation of increasing or decreasing is however really just a special case, applied to partial lifting at each defining angle of zero degrees overhead or ninety degrees over our chest. Because from either position, overhead or over our chest, a point can also be reached where, when employing our full range of motion, pulling now affects an increase in size and so pushing, from that retracted position, tends to diminish the angle of the arc being traced.

As opposed to using our whole arm however an easy way to get a sense for the control of either appendage, as directed by just the musculature of our upper-torso, is by simply reaching back with one hand (either right or left) and then grasping its attached shoulder joint. Because with our forearm immobilized, through holding onto our shoulder, that effectively negates the importance of any sensory feedback from our hand, as our elbow joint now becomes the perceived extremity for that arm. Applying my simple shoulder-grasping technique to a more realistic situation, such as with weightlifting, would then merely entail not extending our focus point of control past our elbows. However since our innate inclination is towards our hands it can take some time getting used to, this sense for the directing of either arm through our shoulders.

But although depicted as the requisite way of consciously controlling either arm it is of course from just trying to improve on our perceiving of this disparity, in our sense of initiating, that invokes the interim increase in the acuity of our spatial discerning, which I define as engaging a dual sensory focus. However because it establishes the basis to the accelerated contortions that our body can be conditioned to perform, which are also very exacting in nature, is the underlying reason for specifically invoking our maintaining of acute shoulder control, rather than our more commonly employed sense of compelling. For it was only after partaking in a routine of deliberately reiterating through a sense of acute shoulder control, the full swing motion of both my forehand and backhand, that I was able to readily get a feel for this alternative to fixed focus-point initiating. But although defined as simply a sense of our apex of manipulation moving outward, as our swing motion unfolds, my insight (expressed as a concise mental concept) is in fact a distilling of a number of presentations on stroke development, from both personal instruction and various forms of media. The idea was then reinforced not only through the enhancing of my own performance, from employing a shifting point of control, but also from various conversations with my brother, an avid tennis player, who describes the concept in a more physical sense as a "full-body swing".

So rather than a single concocted notion, as related to our sport of choice, a dual sensory approach actually extends to encompassing two different assertions, for improving on our emulating of any associated physical contortions. Where on the one hand, albeit unsubstantiated, the presumption being that the same invoking of precise shoulder control, used to constrain our sense of initiating to primarily the musculature of our upper-torso, is also what defines the basis to our exacting sense of accelerated directing, through a shifting apex of manipulation. The other assertion of course being that an increase in the acuity of our spatial discerning can also be compelled by simply trying to get a better feel for this difference in the flexing of either arm, with our focus point of control as sensed from our hand or invoked through our shoulder. And with the related impact, from the accumulated time engaging a dual sensory focus, being in theory what led to the rather sudden increase in the consistency of my tennis strokes.

Originally though it was in a class on sports psychology where I was first introduced to the use of sensory enhancing exercises, as a circuitous method for improving on the incisiveness of our initiating. For the discussion during one session was about the use of physical movement, with the express purpose of invoking an increase in the acuity of our spatial discerning. Although the actual technique elaborated on can be described as a "simplifying" of what is used in Tai Chi. Because instead of a contrived set of complex physical articulations, to try and engage a sensory focus, all mental effort is directed at just maintaining acute muscle control, irrespective of any particular motion used. And so with no specific routine I refer to the mindset of this rather forthright approach, for invoking an increase in the acuity of our spatial discerning, as a "simple" sensory focus. More commonly though, like with Tai Chi, acute muscle control is sustained through the deliberate emulating of an explicit series of motions, hence the name for the particular mindset employed. All of which is to say that I found it rather difficult to maintain acute muscle control, for any extended period of time, therefore I never seriously took up freeform sensory enhancing with its more austere approach, to the issue of improving on the incisiveness of our initiating.

Ultimately though it is our maintaining of acute muscle control, through any type of sensory focus, that defines the basis to our descending sensory pathways allowing for a diminishing in the inherent impedance of our attending ascending neural pathways, thereby improving on the relaying of inner sensory feedback. My use of resistance, through weightlifting, being merely a way of more effectively precipitating the process by employing sensory feedback of a greater perceived intensity; which is in fact reflected through a higher signal frequency as neural sensory information is conveyed more through varying the number of transmission pulses, rather than modulating signal amplitude. The contention however, that increased impedance could potentially decrease response time, is actually based on analysis reflecting the physiological adaptations incurred by our neural activating circuits, which transmit efferent control signals, rather than our ascending sensory pathways, where these changes are attributed to be occurring. For when a motor neuron fires, through assessing the mechanical tension generated from the resulting muscle contraction, a direct numerical correlation can be established with the amplitude and pulse rate of an applied efferent control signal. With afferent sensory information on the other hand only our mind can determine, through its own referencing, the importance of signal frequency and voltage, as caused by an applied stimulus, and so any results, by actual testing, must be derived through some type of subjective association. Although what leads to an increase in the number of variables, any type of analysis must contend with, is the fact that our perception of stretch and tension feedback is closely related to our inherent strength, an attribute based not only on contractile force but also mechanical advantage. And so a random group of test subjects might *not* necessarily follow the trend where a set weight is always considered relatively light, by those who are more robust, while those who are less endowed sense the same resistance as being at least moderately heavy. Therefore in reviewing the basic operation of every cell body, designed primarily for relaying sensory information, particular attention is given to the neural circuitry associated with the triggering of motor neurons, since testing does allow for results that can be readily verified.

Now because of operationally being similar in that each discriminates by triggering just a single output, oftentimes initiated by a multitude of input signals, a neuron (as already noted) can be compared to an electronic gate. Functionally however what distinguishes most neural tissue, from almost every kind digital circuit, is that as reflected through a change in signal frequency the intensity level required, to generate an output, can oftentimes be varied. On a physical level at least that degree of neural reprogramming, which impacts on when a neuron fires, is achieved through simply repeating an explicit series of motions. Whereby from continually engaging the same neural interconnections, through reiterating an specific motion sequence, over time that tends to compel a progressive lowering in the prevailing impedance of the neurons along the circuit in question. This diminishing in the impetus required, to initiate an output, is then what allows a routinely practiced motion sequence to become so integrated that, to perform with a fair degree of proficiently, almost no conscious oversight is needed. The obvious example of course of this physical erudition process occurs early in life when mastering the skill of controlled falling or walking, as it is more commonly called.

But as brought on by any type of learning activity this redefining of operational parameters is not confined to just impacting on the prevailing impedance to triggering an output, as it can also extend to actually altering our brain's neural circuitry. Whereby from simply reiterating an explicit motion sequence, thereby excluding a number of other possibilities, over time that can lead to some neural interconnections being so neglected, from a lack of use, as to cease functioning. On the other hand a routinely repeated motion sequence may also spur the growth of new interconnections between neurons, as a way to further hardwire into active control. So the question is what are the various attributes, related to every learning activity, that can actually be manipulated to increase our rate of neural restructuring. For that would denote, in terms of any exacting physical activity, how to possibly improve on, in a more expeditious manner, our emulating of a particular motion sequence.

Derived then from the same three factors, used for establishing the primary benefit of any exercise routine, my understanding is that our acquisition rate, from any learning activity, is essentially based on intensity, duration and frequency. The difference in this case being that intensity acts as a "catalyst" which tends to diminish the response time required for the integrating process of learning, instead of defining the physiological response of either directly affecting cellular respiration or by impacting on a more anaerobic form of releasing cellular energy. Although it is through increasing the number of times a motion is reiterated and/or by augmenting the intensity of an applied efferent control signal that, with regards to any contorting of our body, a resistance-conditioning routine can actually be used, to incur a faster reprogramming of any associated neural circuitry. Which is to say a physical therapy center is probably the more noted locale where all three attributes (intensity, duration and frequency) are readily employed, as a way to optimize the impact of an applied stimulus.

Unlike with any resistance-conditioning routine however, which a physical therapist might use, most learning activities have no way of consistently maintaining a high level of intensity, at best we are able to control both the duration and frequency of an applied stimulus. Of course in certain exacting physical activities, such as golf and tennis, the tri-factor learning theory does allude to the possibility of employing higher levels of inner sensory feedback. The concern however with using heavier than normal equipment is that, through an "exaggeration" of what are normally very precise efferent control signals, our degree of accuracy, in our emulating of the contortions of our activity of choice, could be detrimentally affected. Consequently why the only way of directly improving on the incisiveness of our initiating is through continually practicing (to perfect) the motions employed by our chosen sport or dance, oftentimes through specific drills that stress just one particular attribute.

In a somewhat similar fashion, as related to affecting the acuity of our spatial discerning, the scope of a dual sensory approach is also constrained to encompassing merely a single attribute. For rather than the actual control of an attached appendage the increased force and displacement feedback, from lifting weights, is primarily intended for just impacting on the neurons that relay afferent sensory information, although not with the usual response of highly selective filtering. Because with a dual sensory focus, as with any sensory enhancing mindset, neural sensory information is employed, at the discretion of our descending sensory pathways, as a mechanism for easing the conveyance (along our ascending sensory pathways) of the resulting stretch and tension feedback, brought on by the contracting of our skeletal musculature. And with the higher signal frequency, brought on by the increased resistance from lifting weights, that should in theory allow for compelling a faster decrease in the inherent impedance of the transmitting neurons, along the enabled ascending sensory pathways. Consequently less time is required for the low levels of force and displacement feedback, which normally traverse our ascending sensory pathways, to be more acutely perceived through an overall enhanced sense of proprioception. That then being my contention which presumes to denote, through the sustaining of acute muscle control, the impact on the relaying of afferent sensory information to our brain and not what a sensory focus does to the other half of our neural control loop, the descending motor pathways, where the actual directing of our skeletal musculature resides.

My presumption though on this supplemental effect of enhancing sensory awareness remains for now mere speculation, since the results from the testing of any technique (claiming to indirectly improve on the incisiveness of our initiating) are rather tenuous in nature. Because how can it be definitively proven that an enhancing in our degree of emulating was in fact caused by the conditioning from employing some type of sensory enhancing mindset. For whether performing a single precise motion or a whole series of exacting physical contortions every practice I have alluded to, for improving on the acuity of our spatial discerning, is essentially mental in nature. And so ascertaining that a particular technique is being employed correctly, if at all, is a matter of contention. Therefore through actually employing, what I have described as a dual a sensory mindset, is the only way to know for sure if this mental technique really works or if it is simply a guise, to entice one into resistance conditioning.

Construed then as merely a form of bilateral sensory information processing a dual sensory focus is in part defined by a left-brain metaphysical construct, described as active control, which attends to the deliberate directing of arms, as controlled primarily by the musculature of our upper-torso. And unless physically forced through a restricting of motion this enabling of acute shoulder control is almost always (at least initially) beset with a tendency, which we need to resist, of our focus point of manipulation shifting back to our hands, thereby returning primary control back to the musculature of our upper-arm. Concurrently of course, along with our left cerebral cortex, the right half of our brain is also engaged in the discerning of inner sensory feedback. However rather than being employed as a spatial recalibrating gauge, as with a specific sensory focus, passive sensing (the contrived metaphysical component of our right cerebral cortex) is instead used for distinguishing the subtle difference in localized intensity between hand and shoulder control. With the inclination here, which we need to resist, being that of not fixating on a single type of directing, either from our upper-arm or upper-torso, thereby losing the bilateral distinctness of a dual sensory mindset. For although acute muscle control is more readily sustained through engaging a specific sensory focus, as exertion levels increase, a singular mindset is more susceptible to being compelled into becoming a high-intensity specific focus; thereby effectively reducing passive sensing to being, in terms of inner sensory feedback, merely a means of gauging physical exertion.

Now although invoking an interim increase in the acuity of our spatial discerning is not always easy, as distractions abound, my use of a dual sensory focus is at least tangibly based on just consciously differentiating between our focus point of control as centered on our hands or invoked through our shoulders. Because only several weeks of mental technique refining were required, through twice a week lifting sessions, for me to initially assess that I had achieved a level of success, from employing a dual sensory approach. With the evidence being reflected, as mentioned earlier, by the rather sudden improvement in the consistency of my racket head making contact with the ball, thereby reducing the number of unforced errors I made while playing tennis. For I had seemingly attained an increase in localized kinesthetic awareness where an acute sense of shoulder control, which I had already developed a few years earlier, was no longer a transitory sensation. Because for over ten years, during which I employed a dual sensory approach, I was able to retain a degree of spatial cognizance that before was usually attained only after about a half-hour of warm-up practice and then was just temporary. Although it was only after a few months, from having acquired a fuller appreciation of all the physical benefits gained from employing a dual sensory focus, that I initially considered writing a book to describe my mental technique, as applied to a concise lifting routine. Another ten years would pass however before I actually made a concerted effort to try and describe a dual sensory approach, in terms of both its physical and mental constraints. Because how does one begin to explain that a concise lifting routine needs to be done in such a way that essentially looks like ordinary weightlifting, except maybe a little slower?

Thus the reason for opening with a discussion on the structure of our brain as defined through the difference, in terms of sensory information processing, between our left and right cerebral cortex. Although rather than coming straight-out and trying to describe passive sensing and active control, the two contrived metaphysical components which denote the discerning of our inner sense of touch by either side of our brain. Instead because it made for a more compelling example a visual context was first considered to define this generalized distinction in the evaluating of sensory information, by each hemispheric lobe of our cerebrum. Hopefully that provided at least the basis for an understanding where, even if essentially done the same way, a dual sensory approach is considered a mental activity, with its underlying effect being more far reaching than just maintaining a high degree of muscle tone. Of course the reason for this restricting on our degree of physical development is because the level of resistance we are able to employ, and still engage a dual sensory focus, is only a fraction (about three-fourths) of what would be considered more ideal, in terms of developing strength.

Finally to close out this chapter the difference will now be considered between what I call physical forcing, where the prime mover employed is determined through primarily the restricting of motion, and mental directing, where only our mind is used to try and isolate a particular muscle group. Initially however a barbell will be employed for just distinguishing between the physical forcing of control, either through our shoulders or towards either extremity. Because with a barbell the mere positioning of our hands can act as the physical constraint that determines which particular muscle group (of our upper-arm or upper-torso) will be primarily employed. For the effect of grasping a barbell, with our hands very close together, is that we effectively restrict any movement by either shoulder; thus extending our elbows through their full range of motion and so, depending on the exercise, either our biceps or triceps do most of the work. A very wide grip, on the other hand, tends to limit the flexing of either elbow joint, in effect forcing our shoulders through a more complete arc of its extended range of motion; thereby more actively engaging the musculature of our upper-torso. With a barbell then by simply varying the distance between our hands we are able to designate which similar function muscle group, within upper-arm or upper-torso, will be primarily affected from the exercise employed.

Between those two extremes however of physically forcing control to either our hands or through our shoulders there is also a neutral position of no particular emphasis and so any muscle isolation, if desired, must be developed through conscious selection. Normally that interval, where the articulations of our elbow and shoulder are about equal in range of motion, is most conveniently set at slightly greater than the width of our back. Therefore to more readily enable a dual sensory focus the distance maintained, between our hands, should be at that personally defined spacing where it is relatively easy to alternate between primarily elbow flexing and a sense of directing, as initiated through our shoulders. And with our perceiving of that subtle disparity, between our two basic forms of arm control, being what extends our use of passive sensing beyond spatial recalibrating, to essentially embody the right brain aspect of a dual sensory focus.

At first it may seem a little involved but that is of course intentional as the express purpose is to keep one's mind actively engaged, while performing a relatively simple exercise routine. Understanding how to enable a dual sensory focus is however the easy part, as getting a sense of what to "feel" for just takes a little experimenting. The difficult part with this approach, as with every other method of sensory enhancing, is in establishing the basis for a readily enabled mental disposition and not letting the activity be reduced to simply its physical attributes. For maintaining acute muscle control, through any kind of sensory mindset, requires a fair degree of effort. However adding to the resolution needed, with a dual sensory focus, is the fact that the four motions involved are so basic each can be done with almost no consciousness oversight. Naturally any lack of mental effort from doing the four exercises, defining a dual sensory approach, is somewhat negated by increased resistance, which usually compels us to try and engage a sensory moderating mindset. On the plus side is the fact that because of consisting of only eight to ten repetitions the sustained interval of time, for invoking an increase in the acuity of our spatial discerning, is relatively transitory in nature.

Successfully maintaining acute muscle control, through a dual sensory focus, can then be envisioned as a mental balancing act where, up to a point, the greater the resistance the more effective the stimulus for improving on the incisiveness of our initiating. Therefore in the next chapter, after describing the four exercise motions and a few alternatives for each one, the discussion shifts to other issues of consequence, as for example grip tension and breathing. Because not just the aforementioned related attributes (of grip tension and breathing) as any number of unrelated issues are also oftentimes employed, as a means to tip the scales on our engaging of a dual sensory focus.

Chapter 3

The Program

Of course as already denoted, in terms of strictly its overt manifestation, a dual sensory approach is in fact just a concise four-exercise lifting routine, for stressing the various musculature of our upper-body. From the introduction and last two chapters however, although somewhat abstract and oversimplified, my detailing should have allowed for at least a working understanding of how to effectively enable the related mental disposition, defined as simply a dual sensory mindset. But because of being somewhat abstract and oversimplified, before discussing the aforementioned exercises, an attempt at further clarification will be endeavored.

The engaging of a sensory focus, to maintain acute muscle control, is then envisioned as not just a single fixed mindset but a more encompassing mental template, whose variations embrace at least three marginally distinct ways of positively impacting on the incisiveness of our initiating. And so from primarily the practice of Tai Chi we have our first related disposition, defined as a specific sensory focus. Next we have a dual sensory mindset, from a differentiating approach to weightlifting; and finally a demeanor described as a simple sensory focus, from partaking in freeform sensory enhancing. Now rather than engaging in a direct comparison, to try and establish a sense for the subtle disparity denoting the difference between an explicit sensory and a dual sensory mindset, instead I initially endeavored to assess the more encompassing nature of just a specific focus, irrespective of disposition. Although to actually do all of the above I first applied the two-brain theory, based on a contrast in hemispheric processing. From there, as related to its binary fracturing, I extrapolated on function and concocted the notion of two metaphysical components, passive sensing and active control, to reflect the difference in our discerning of inner sensory feedback by each hemispheric lobe of our cerebrum. The idea of bilateral sensory information processing was then extended to encompass the notion where each hemispheric center is able to analyze the transduced sensory stimuli, from any one our five senses, in either relative isolation or through close coordination between our left and right cerebral cortex. And so in the context of stretch and tension feedback this concept, presuming on operational interface, was denoted through either a predominately left-brain specific focus, employing just active control, or an actively interfacing whole brain sensory mindset, albeit oftentimes singular in disposition. But what actually defines the basis to where the difference lies, in the utilization of our mental faculties, between a specific focus directed at simply emulating a previously integrated motion sequence and a more precision oriented sensory mindset, consciously reflected through an invoked increase in the acuity of our spatial discerning?

I of course attribute this distinction, between engaging just active control and maintaining acute muscle control, as essentially a consequence of our shifting (either consciously or reflexively) to an inherent mindset, highly conducive to a complex process referred to simply as learning. Where physiologically what defines any learning activity, either physical or purely cerebral, is in being a stimulus for affecting the coherent restructuring of certain neural networks and not just of our brain, as the possibilities of impacting on neural integration really extended to every part of our nervous system. And so our maintaining of acute muscle control is then viewed, in terms of its overall purpose, as simply a physical erudition process that although not exclusively is usually engaged through a specific sensory focus, directed at either a singular explicit motion or a whole series of exacting contortions.

Instead of neural recalibrating however, as with a specific mindset, a dual sensory focus extends on our use of passive sensing to encompass its more rudimentary ability of differentiating between different degrees of intensity, as related to a particular sensory stimulus. Although rather than simply conveying an overall sensation, commonly referred to as our perceived degree of exertion, instead stretch and tension feedback is acutely discerned for defining the more localized difference in stress between the directing of our arms by primarily the musculature of either our upper-arm or upper-torso. Because by engaging in perceiving this subtle disparity, between hand and shoulder control, is what in theory allows for invoking an increase in the acuity of our spatial discerning, with no real emphasis on the motion being emulated. Compared to a singular mindset however the real advantage of a dual sensory focus being that, at the increased intensity of resistance conditioning, we are less likely to defer to our innate tendency of engaging in sensory moderating. And for those who participate in some sort of exacting physical activity an additional benefit being that, compared to a specific focus, a more ambiguous mindset reduces the degree of neural integration, generally related to any type of deliberate emulating. Implying that engaging a dual sensory focus is then one way of diminishing, from the lifting exercises performed, any possible adverse effect that might impact on an already fine-tuned kinesthetic memorization of the motions used in one's activity of choice.

But although consisting of just a concise four-exercise lifting routine it is because of effectively employing all related sets of skeletal musculature of significance, in both our arms and upper torso, that a dual sensory approach essentially defines a complete upper-body workout. And even if invoking a differentiating sensory mindset tends to limit the amount of weight we are able to lift, and still maintain acute muscle control, usually it is more than adequate since skilled athletes employ precision power based more on timing and speed of movement, rather than sheer brute strength. With the term adequate in this case applying to those individuals, like myself, whose goal is merely optimal fitness and so are not aspiring to perform at a level that, to try and attain a competitive edge, normally requires more intense training. That then being my exclusionary disclaimer regarding professional athletes, having really no experience in that field of endeavor.

I do however understand the demands placed on the recreational athlete because, although having played earlier, since the latter part of nineteen eighty-seven my sport of choice has been singles tennis, which I managed to play on a relatively consistent basis for the next twelve years. Precipitated by overuse however an early injury is what led to a number of upper-body resistance-conditioning exercises being initially employed, through simply maintaining muscle tone, as a way of reducing the chance of incurring another injury. And as they had been since nineteen seventy-eight, from primarily running, my legs (of the lower half of my body) were used to augment my aerobic capacity, thereby endowing me with at least the fitness required to compete at any sport but especially one so physically demanding as singles tennis. And so through developing both strength and stamina, the two primary physical conditioning alternatives, I was able to effectively employ all related sets of skeletal musculature of significance for controlling both my arms and legs, thus defining almost a complete workout.

The reason then for me not normally engaging in any extensive lower-body resistance conditioning, except possibly after an extended layoff, is because of running being such an effective stimulus, on all leg and lower back muscles, it makes any additional exercises somewhat redundant. For the probable increase in contractile force, acquired from partaking in a series of lower-body resistance-conditioning exercises, is now viewed as a comparatively minor physiological benefit, since running conveys a similar albeit weaker response. Although with my emphasis of always looking for an incline to ascend even that slight deficiency, in developing strength, is somewhat compensated for by the increased resistance to motion, from negotiating an incline. Additionally running uphill also allows for inducing an augmenting in our aerobic capacity at a reduced level of structural stress compared to the pace required, from running on level ground, to achieve a similar degree of intensity. All of which is to say that for most people the additional calories burned is probably the main benefit incurred from, compared to partaking in just running, all the effort expended engaging in a series of explicit leg strengthening exercises. Of course to some individuals that is really not an issue, since initially their primary goal for exercising is just losing weight. Personally I advocate partaking in a physical activity based more on skill, such as golf or tennis, where there really is more room for expanding on the possibilities, compared to the rather austere nature of most means for increasing either strength or stamina. Also because of the practice of most competitive activities of skill being less intense, than engaging in weightlifting, in effect that means a higher percentage of fat is actually used as an energy source, to drive cellular respiration.

Similar to running then my rationale for only doing four upper-body resistance-conditioning exercises is also based on the idea that, from any additional lifting, there is a rather significant diminishing in our body's adaptation response, in terms of the anatomical enhancing being induced. And so because simply maintaining an acceptable level of fitness doesn't really require an inordinate amount of effort is the reason, as I see it, why most books on implementing the overload principle were conceived with the notion of appealing to our more competitive nature. For if one's goal, realistic or not, is to compete in an extreme sport, such as bodybuilding or power lifting, then a rather comprehensive regimen of some form of resistance conditioning is usually called for, to more effectively achieve one's full potential. However with most of us not engaged in the exhibition of our physical prowess, to the point of entering into some type of sanctioned competition, that means fully adhering to any of the associated resistance-conditioning programs is really not required. Because in terms of impacting the musculature of our upper-body a majority of the gains, from any extensive workout, can be achieved from a routine consisting of just four lifting exercises.

So rather than the more conventional approach of trying to employ all pertinent sets of skeletal musculature, irrespective of redundancy, my assessment is instead about the optimizing of physical effort, through an understanding of both physiology and the concept described here simply as our body's adaptation response. And so from the multitude of exercises available, in terms of strictly physiology, it is simply a case of establishing just what exactly is needed to effectively engage all the prime movers employed in affecting any movement we initiate and not be overly redundant. A bit more inexplicable however is the related notion of our body's adaptation response, to any kind physical stress, and so a wider range of interpretation exists for denoting just what exactly would be considered optimal, in terms of an actual exercise routine. Although as defined through the three impacting factors of intensity, duration and frequency the various adaptations incurred, from any kind of exercise routine, can be readily assessed by measuring the difference in performance over a set period of time, as related to usually just one of the three attributes of fitness be it strength, speed or stamina. My conclusions regarding our body's adaptation response are then essentially an encapsulating of a number of studies that, through correlating the three factors to a particular routine, gauged the extent of a particular benefit incurred, as related to the concept of diminishing returns.

Now expanding on an oft-used visual analogy, citing a bull in a china shop, the concept of diminishing returns can be seen as defining a hypothetical demarcation point where, because of the number of items having been destroyed, there is a significant reduction in the amount of damage caused by any additional kicking. Applied to fitness the notion of diminishing returns is then used for establishing when an exercise, for developing either strength or stamina, ceases to have a corresponding adaptation response, in terms of conferring some sort of anatomical enhancing. Although it would appear, from the current wave of fitness advertising, that this transition point has been relegated to merely an insignificant juncture for establishing when the burning of calories finally becomes the main benefit incurred, from extending the duration of a promoted activity. Of course with any competitive activity of a primarily physical nature, since all the top athletes have about the same genetic predisposition, the stress of additional conditioning is oftentimes the determining factor in how well one does against the competition. From a standpoint of strictly optimal conditioning however since any advantage gained is usually not exploited, which would at least justify the extra effort, doing anything beyond the prescribed routine is probably an expenditure that could be better utilized, especially if we participate in a physical activity based more on skill.

But while effectively stressing all pertinent sets of skeletal musculature for controlling my arms and legs this tandem of a four-exercise lifting program and running was also described as *not* fully conforming to the requirements of what defines a complete workout. For a core muscle group, specifically the set layered across my stomach, is unaffected by either running or the aforementioned four exercises. On the other hand, as the antagonist to my abdominal muscles, the musculature of my lower back is effectively engaged during both running and weightlifting. And so anatomically speaking the reason for my doing some sort of abdominal resistance-conditioning exercise is to establish a balance in strength with the opposing muscle groups of my lower back. As a key to preventing injuries is through maintaining symmetry in strength development and so a defining aspect of any thorough lifting program is in being denoted by complementary or offsetting exercises that effectively employ both contrary sets of skeletal musculature, along the plane of motion in question.

Of course also related to this concept of injury prevention is the reason that I continued adhering to a concise upper-body resistance-conditioning program, even though having fully recovered from the physical impairment caused by my initial tennis related injury. Because like most exacting physical activities tennis is very asymmetric in terms of how, from continually contorting our body, the resulting physical stress impacts on our skeletal musculature. Where over the long-term this constrained utilization, from just reiterating the particular motions related to our activity of choice, is what leads to the problems associated with an imbalance in muscle development. Initially however, due to a lack of conditioning, asymmetric muscle usage is what oftentimes allows for overuse to be a primary cause, as to how injuries are often incurred. Irrespective though of its injury preventing benefits, through symmetrical muscle development, most of us who do strive to excel at the practice of resistance conditioning usually manage, at some time or another, to physically damage at least one of the four components, defining our body's lever system.

Affecting then both novice and veteran the reason as I see it, as the underlying cause of most lifting injuries, is because of what it takes for an optimal invoking of our body's physical ability, in terms of overcoming a set impedance. For ultimately the full potential of our body's lever system, as related to how much weight we are able to lift, is derived from not only maximizing the contractile force our muscles are able to generate, as it is also related to how quickly the activity of contracting occurs. My evidence for this presumption, on essentially the importance of acceleration, is most impressively displayed in the extreme sport of power lifting where what is usually employed, to overcome a set impedance, are both sheer strength and an ability to engage in rapid movement. Although what actually allows us to move so fast is only in part based on the celerity of contracting by our muscles because, as with most vertebrae, our mechanical lever system is in fact designed for "motion multiplying" as it is called. This adeptness of ours, at quickly contorting our arms and legs, is then of course employed at every level of impedance, with golf and tennis each being an example of a sport at the low end of the resistance scale.

Versus overuse however, where problems tend occur with activities of low impedance, the main detriment at the other end of the resistance scale is in the persuasiveness of over-stress injuries. My guess being that of the multitude who have ever partaken, in some form of resistance conditioning, most probably had a very limited understanding of how their body's mechanical lever system actually operates, consequently they had no idea that the cost of accelerated motion is derived from a multiplying of applied force. Essentially what that means is the prime mover employed may initially need to generate, with a pushing exercise, a combined contractile force extending from three to over five times the inherent gravitational force, exerted by the attending implement of impedance. (With a pulling exercise, compelled by primarily the musculature of our upper-torso, just the opposite occurs as increased force is needed the closer the implement of impedance gets to our body.) The real concern however, with the practice of overload conditioning, is actually in the elevated levels of physical stress placed on the associated components of our lever system, from the sheer amount of force conveyed through the contracting our skeletal musculature. Of course the way to reduce the risk of incurring an injury is by simply lifting less weight but how can there still be an optimizing of the anatomical enhancing incurred by our body, through maximizing the degree of effort needed against a set impedance?

Well with an aerobic exercise the easiest way to affect an increase in our perception of physical intensity is by just setting a faster pace, although altering resistance to motion (whenever possible) is also an effective way to vary the degree of effort required. For even a slight increase in impedance can so significantly augment our sense of the incurred physical stress that we are forced to slow down, sometimes drastically. On the other hand, with the already augmented impedance of a muscle strengthening exercise, what I perceived was a reverse correlation between pace of movement and how that affected how much effort I was exerting. Because contrary to what happens with an aerobic exercise, where slowing down tends to diminish our sense of the incurred physical stress, what I sensed from lifting any weight considered at least moderately heavy was that, compared to an accelerated motion, deliberate movement significantly increased the amount of effort required. Earlier of course, in the first chapter "Passive Sensing", this seemingly counterintuitive consequence, related to the degree of physical effort required, was described as simply the inverse effect of high-resistance. And with the longer duration of a deliberate pace, versus a faster motion, being the underlying cause (over the relatively minute interval of time during which it actually applies) for this contrary effect of augmented impedance from lifting against resistance. As an inherent structural design, meant for quickly accelerating our limbs, is also what defines the basis to my contention that speed, and not brute strength, is the real source of our physical prowess. Newton's first law of motion is however what denotes the scientific underpinning as to the actual cause of this inverse effect of high-resistance; for lifting slowly means that in effect the force, which must be continuously overcome, is the initial inertia of a body at rest. But rather than our more complex lever system, though which we initiate any contorting of body, instead the simpler mechanics of a seesaw will be employed, as a means to assess the connection between the aforementioned "motion multiplying" and its "multiplying of force" requirement. For although appearing seemingly disparate functionally however the only thing that really distinguishes our body's lever system, from the average seesaw, is in its increased complexity and so defining the actual dynamics is a more involved process.

Now since any weight placed on either end would have tended to create, at the other end, an upward force equal in magnitude essentially that means the pivot point was in the middle of the board of almost every seesaw I ever rode on. With the implication being that pairs of individuals, who partake in riding on these equilibrium based seesaws, should be pretty close to being about the same weight. Because with a child and an adult, where the disparity in mass is oftentimes quite significant, the average seesaw can be rather limiting since the lighter youth spends most of the time up in the air, with the heavier adult controlling all movement. To compensate for that possibility (of an imbalance in weight) some seesaws allow the board to be repositioned along the fulcrum; in effect putting the child a greater distance from the pivot point than the adult, who is moved closer in. A longer lever then allows the lesser gravitational force of the adolescent, on the extended end of the board, to offset the adult on the other side. The trade-off being that the child has to travel a greater distance, to displace the heavier adult over a shorter interval.

Now in fact having many practical applications, with a crowbar being just one example of a simple tool used for translating movement into increased force or pressure, from the child's perspective on the seesaw the lever system employed is actually called a force multiplier. Of course if our body's lever system had been predominately designed as a force multiplier that would have in theory given us an ability to lift almost anything previously considered way too heavy. Although because of the constraints imposed on our lever system the set interval, any object could actually be raised, would be rather insignificant. However since we are able to affect, from rather minute changes in interlacing displacement, a comparatively high degree of spatial displacing in effect that means the primary articulations of our body are in fact designed more from the perspective of the heavier of the two individuals on the seesaw. For the adult, who sits closer in, moves very little as the child, on the other side of the board, goes way up and down. But because of the elapsed time being the same for both the shorter distance, covered by the adult, and the much larger interval, traversed by the youth, in effect that means the child must travel faster than the adult. The advantage gained here then, although not really exploited, is in the form of acceleration; consequently why in terms of the adult, on short end of the board, the type of lever system employed is called a motion multiplier. And with the cost of faster movement being of course the greater force, from the increased mass of adult, needed to offset a much smaller mass, the lighter child, dependent on the ratio of the distances (from the pivot point) of each opposing end of the lever being employed.

Unlike with the simplistic operation of most seesaws however, whatever their configuration, any contorting we initiate is a more complex process with the effective leverage distance actually varying with the changing angle, through the flexing of either our arms or legs. And so instead of being set at a fixed amount, as with a seesaw, due to the nature of the connection between muscle and bone the applied force required will increase or decrease, depending on the action being performed (pushing out or pulling in). In the extreme, as when doing a deep-knee bend, that can of course mean an augmenting, in the amount of contractile force needed, from between three to over five times what the force of gravity places on the object we decide to pick up, with our legs in this case. With almost every exacting physical activity however the implement used is relatively light and so the resulting stress placed on our lever system, from correctly employing said implement, is normally by itself not the actual cause of most injuries incurred. On the other hand, as a way of increasing the contractile force of any number of muscle groups, with overload conditioning the whole idea is to place an inordinate amount of stress on our body's mechanical lever system. And although this structural design integrating muscle, bone, ligament and tendon is an engineering marvel of nature it is not perfect, as attested to by the sheer number of injuries incurred from partaking in the practice resistance conditioning. Now one reason for that being because with almost every means of expeditiously developing strength, due to a disparity in our adaptation response, the contractile force our muscles are able to generate can increase so quickly other parts our lever system may actually be jeopardized, because of not being able to readily adapt.

Based then on a correlation, between blood flow and the rate of cellular growth or repair, the contention being that ligaments and tendons are more prone to injury, compared to muscle and bone. Because the more blood that passes through a particular area means more nutrition is available, thus allowing for either faster healing or proliferation to occur. And so with the large number of blood vessels, infusing our muscles and bones, that implies those two components of our body's lever system adapt rather quickly to the effects of physical stress. Ligaments and tendons, on the other hand, are not as permeated with blood vessels and so as a consequence these supporting structures have a slower adaptation response to any augmenting in workload, defined here through increasing impedance to motion. The concern then being that, after the first few weeks of resistance conditioning, our muscles seem to rather expeditiously give us a "feeling" of being able to handle more weight, after every set increase in impedance to motion. Attending connective tissue however, with its restricted circulation, may still be adapting to the last increase in the amount being lifted. And so by too hastily implementing the overload principle, and adding more weight, we increase the probability of straining a ligament or tendon, thus a common injury sustained by those initially engaging in some form of resistance conditioning. As more experienced weightlifters, through effective physical development and an overly effective repressing of inner sensory feedback, extend the possibilities to damaging any one to all four components defining their body's lever system.

But besides reducing the chance of incurring an injury lifting less weight also allows for more readily maintaining deliberate movement, the physical attribute most often employed as a means of concurrently inducing an increase in the acuity of our spatial discerning. Which is of course why, in addition to localized differentiating, a dual sensory focus also encompasses the meticulous emulating of movement, in our effort to maintain acute muscle control. In terms of strictly physical benefits however, compared to a faster motion, the advantage of a deliberate pace is of course reflected in the related increase in our perception of physical effort, from simply slowing down the lifting process. Essentially implying that from what is normally incurred by lifting more weight can also be attained, through merely employing a more leisurely pace. Although from what I have seen it is only the more experienced bodybuilders who tend to openly exploit, what I refer to as the inverse effect of high resistance. But enough conjecture about the advantage of deliberate lifting as it is time to define the basis to the four exercises, mentioned at the beginning of this chapter, that embody the essence of a dual sensory approach.

Initially then it was just the direction in which effort must exerted, through either pushing out or pulling in, that was the only criteria for establishing some type of classification distinction between all the various lifting motions, for strengthening or simply toning our upper-body. Because the design of our body's lever system is such that, although functionally denoted as a complementary tandem, the real differentiation in our use comes from the fact that each aspect (of either tandem) is actually defined by at least two opposing sets of skeletal musculature. However because of the operational scheme employed that means besides the distinction of either being a pushing-out or pulling-in motion a further refining can be established by restricting muscle usage to primarily a single locale, within our upper-arm or upper-torso. Finally, as briefly mentioned in the last chapter, there was a denoting of specific angles of exertion where just one (or the other) similar function upper-torso muscle group was compelled into being the prime mover. And so through extending the implement of resistance straight overhead, with a wide grip, our shoulder muscles or deltoids would be primarily employed, while at best our chest muscles or pectorals are engaged in just static support. Of course at the other defining angle, straight over our chest, the situation is reversed with our pectorals now the prime mover, as our deltoids are relegated to providing merely static support. One constraint however being that when using free-weights doing any type of chest exercise, which involves pushing, would initially require lying on our back as that directs the force vector of gravity through our arms and not at a right angle, as when standing.

But by being described as defining points of isolation in effect that means by shifting just a few degrees from either position, straight overhead or straight over our chest, a more dynamic interaction is enabled between both upper-torso muscle groups, our delts and pecs. And so as a way to increase muscle definition, in both shoulders and chest, serious bodybuilders will oftentimes exploit other possible angles of exertion, besides the overhead and over-chest position. However since three sets of ten repetitions has been defined as what is considered optimal, for stressing a particular muscle group, albeit sparse only two distinct lifting activities are really needed to encompass the function of pushing, in regards to denoting a thorough routine for either strengthening or simply toning our upper-torso. With my particular preference being, in terms of pushing exercises, the bench press for engaging my pectoral muscles and the military or overhead press to work my deltoids.

Now to complement the various sets of skeletal musculature, used for extending either upper-body appendage, we would need to engage a number of opposing sets of skeletal musculature, employed in the withdrawing of either arm. Although a single large back muscle, the latissmus dorsi, is really the only prime mover employed in upper-torso pulling; since all other muscle groups, which assist in the retracting of either arm, are at least enabled through static support, irrespective of the particular exercise. To maintain symmetry however rather than a single lifting activity two distinct pulling motions will be employed, at the same offsetting angles of exertion as defined for pushing. In this case my particular preference being, in terms of pulling exercises, the lat pull-down and bent-over row.

Although instead of what I actually do, which has yet to be considered, I will continue to designate each exercise as simply a function, either pushing or pulling, as related to a particular spatial orientation. For referencing however "chest push" refers specifically to a bench press exercise, "chest pull" to a bent-over row, "overhead push" to a military press and "overhead pull" to a lat-pull down. Of course as applied to a dual sensory approach each term (either "push" or "pull") is used as merely descriptive indicator for designating direction. Because our sense of control, with a dual sensory focus, should extend from our shoulders and be perceived as an "arc-tracing" sensation and not our more ingrained sense of just elbow-bending, usually invoked through our compelling of either a "pushing" or "pulling" motion.

Now it may appear that I have neglected our arm muscles, as no separate set of exercises will be considered to specifically develop either our biceps or triceps. However under the setup constraints of a dual sensory approach, although not the prime mover in any single exercise, the musculature of each upper-arm is adequately engaged by being employed twice (albeit secondarily) based just on function, regardless of any location specified. This inclusive utilization of our biceps and triceps is then of course the reason why, through actually a variety of exercises, the four lifting motions just discussed essentially define a thorough routine, for either strengthening or simply toning our upper-body. As the basis however to any comprehensive overload-conditioning program a great deal has already been detailed (in both books and magazines) about not only the initial setup constraints, to safely do each aforementioned lifting exercise, but also the numerous options and variations, related to each particular lifting motion. (My definition of an option being a shift in body position and/or physically changing the apparatus used to possibly impact on static muscle support, although it has almost no effect on how the prime mover is actually being employed. With a variation on the other hand, through a shift in body position and/or physically changing the apparatus used, there is some kind of impact on how the prime mover is being employed, static support however is not necessarily affected.) And so with that wealth of information available, on the finer points of lifting, instead of being redundant and also detailing how to do each exercise the following discussion will be restricted to a number of options and variations, which I deem of significance. Finally to close out this chapter the more potent of the many detractors to maintaining a dual sensory focus will be assessed.

Selected then merely for ease of discussion the first exercise to be considered is the chest push that, in terms of free-weights, means initially positioning by lying on our back, usually on a bench. The other chest exercise, when free-weights are involved, also requires a ninety-degree rotation of our body from the upright position although the direction is now clockwise which, if we happen to be standing, simply requires bending over at the waist. As related to the aforementioned free-weight exercises however this restricting on our physical positioning is no longer such a defining constraint as the widespread availability of fitness machines has meant that all four lifting motions can oftentimes be performed, while actually sitting upright in some chair-like apparatus. But lying with our back on a bench, usually with supports for holding the object of resistance to be pushed against, is the traditional way of engaging, depending on the distance maintained between our hands, either the pectoral muscles contained within our upper-torso or the triceps muscles of our upper-arm.

Now an alternative to a barbell is employing a set of dumbbells, although that effectively removes the stability provided by a physical connection between our hands. And so because of the increased muscle control needed, to maintain each arm as an unsupported projection, the amount of weight we are able to lift, when using a set of dumbbells, is usually less than what a barbell would allow for irrespective of our particular disposition. At the other extreme however, as related to maintaining proper lifting form, are a number of the aforementioned mechanical apparatus; in this case those specifically directed at strengthening our upper-torso. Because of all the various types of exercise machines available many are explicitly designed to have a very limited range of motion and so stability is even less a point of contention, than with a barbell. Other mechanical apparatus however, such as certain cable designs, are not as restrictive in the constraining of any superficial movement. The advantage though of almost every type of exercise machine is in generally being safer than free-weights and with the range of motion limitations, which many incorporate, forcing one to maintain proper lifting form. My one minor compliant being that because movement is so constrained, with certain types of exercise machines, maintaining balance (a real-life situation) is not a point of emphasis, as it is most of the time when free-weights are employed.

But lacking any of the specific equipment needed, for resistance conditioning of any kind, the chest push stands out as the only one of the four exercises, which is easily done through its converse implementation commonly known as pushups. Because the problem with an overhead pushing exercise being that, when our body is the implement of impedance, the initial setup entails having to do a handstand, difficult enough for most of us much less actually trying a handstand pushup. And with the body-as-resistance option, for either pulling exercise, the limitation being that both require an elevated bar or something fixed for our hands to grasp, so our body can be pulled up; thus neither setup is really equipment free. The reason then, as I see it, why the chest-push and the overhead pull are usually the only alternatives discussed, where our body is the implement of impedance, is because of the converse option of the chest-pull being impractical and that of the overhead push being next to impossible. Due to my weight however, which severely restricts the number of repetitions I am able to do, my preferred alternative with the second exercise, the overhead pull, being an exercise machine of the lat-pull variety. Although there are now mechanical apparatus that, by partially compensating for our body weight, allow us to actually change the set impedance worked against, when doing either pull-ups (with our hands far apart) or chin-ups (with our hands close together).

Now usually deemed of minor consequence another common variation, applicable to almost every overhead exercise, is the physical situating of the object of resistance either in front or behind our head. And so the reason for noting this difference, in initial arm position, is then not so much about how it impacts on muscle development but because doing behind my head pull-downs lead to problems, as expressed through physical pain, with my serving motion in tennis. For only after I stopped alternating, and just did in front pull-downs, was there a resolution to the severe discomfort I incurred while serving. My example then illustrates that sometimes a restricting or modifying of an exercise may be required since, as related to our sport of choice, a particular motion involved doesn't quite suit our unique body mechanics. Although of the variety of lifting activities possible, where a dual sensory focus can be readily engaged, the overhead pull is the only one I see with any cause for concern, in terms of all the variations related to each particular lifting motion. As for all the different options available, where the prime mover employed is relatively unaffected, it is just with the last two exercises, where static support is a potential issue.

The concern with the third exercise, the chest-pull, then being that the initial setup can entail flexing our body ninety-degrees at the waist, as a way of keeping the force vector inline with the positioning of either arm. Now the advantage of bending over is that although isometrically it engages our lower-back muscles in very actively supporting our upper-body. The danger of course lies in the extreme angle of support and the additional stress that places on our body, from contorting to form a right angle. Therefore those with lower-back related issues should probably, as an alternative to a bent-over row, use a chest-pull machine that employs some type of upper-body support, in lieu of directly stressing one's spine. Or another way of doing a chest-pull exercise, which doesn't require bending over, is on a bench that besides allowing one to lie face down on has the freedom, between its legs, to move a barbell up and down.

The last exercise is then the overhead push, which is of course similar to an overhead pulling motion in also oftentimes allowing for the variation of being done with the object of resistance either in front or behind our head. And because of not having incurred any related problems, with my sport of choice, I would usually lift both ways, in front and behind my head, through alternating after every repetition. Now the one option of significance sometimes allowed for, with both free-weights and machine, is that of sitting in a chair-like apparatus which may provide additional back support.

So although not exactly conforming to the resistance aspect of the overload conditioning theory, defining the constraints on the amount weight that one should attempt to lift. I do believe in adhering to the repetition series proven to elicit the optimal adaptation response, even if in practice I would actually first do an additional set of each exercise. Now whether that frequency series of four sets of ten repetitions is the most effective for enhancing neural sensitivity is of course open to debate; however with really no other viable alternative I have always followed traditional practice, in terms of my core workout. The reason though for my initially doing a separate set of each exercise is because when done deliberately, through almost full extension, the motions make for an effective combined stretching and warm-up routine. This approach to weightlifting is then unlike my more conventional pre-activity routine of explicit stretching exercises, usually done before playing tennis or engaging in my aerobic activity of choice (either walking or running).

The final aspect to be considered is then the notion of an ideal exercise sequence, oftentimes advocated by very specialized regimens on bodybuilding. I however in terms of sensory enhancing don't perceive any particular routine as having an advantage over any other set practice. My only stipulation would be to alternate between pushing and pulling exercises, since that allows functionally similar musculature more recovery time. Personally I like starting with the overhead pull although oftentimes when it was crowded at my local fitness center that wasn't always possible without waiting and so instead, depending on availability, I would do one of the other three exercises. For when it comes to working out I like to maintain a certain pace, regardless of any set routine. I must however contend with a habit we all inherently have, at least to a certain degree, of once developing a set practice of not wanting to deviate from it. What I became aware of though was that the mere anticipating equipment availability made me anxious, since it is such a hit-or-miss affair when lifting at a public place. Therefore when I was at a communal locality that was busy, to minimize my duress as a diversion, I would try not to dwell on the prospect of getting to do my preferred lifting sequence, which was usually enough to alleviate my concern.

The reason though for mentioning what exactly tends to disrupt my concentration is because any number of detractors can act as the impetus, for redirecting our sensory focus. And not just through shifting to a general mindset, whose bilateral disposition actually incorporates a secondary diversion, but by engaging a high-intensity specific focus, as a way to effectively block all peripheral intrusions. Although the actual mechanism oftentimes employed, for our invoking of a sensory suppressing mindset, being any one if not all three attributes, reflecting some aspect of the lifting process. And as already mentioned, at the end of the last chapter, breathing and grip tension being two of the more compelling of the aforementioned attributes. Compared to grip tension however, which is directly related to the act of lifting, breathing is seen as a more indirect attribute, with its persuasive influence being employed by any number of activities both physical and strictly mental. The third detractor, also inherently part of the lifting process, is defined as simply extending our elbow joint (of either arm) to the lockout position.

But in spite of being an indirect attribute breathing is probably the most compelling of the three at redirecting our mindset, in part because of being so easy to monitor and control. Which isn't meant to imply that the conscious regulating of our lung fluctuations is in every way detrimental to a dual sensory approach, as proper breathing technique is a habit well worth acquiring. And with so many books on Yoga already explaining how to "belly breath", as the practice is commonly called, I won't elaborate any further. I will however allude to belly breathing as being similar to a dual sensory focus, since initially either technique is relatively easy to learn. Likewise the difficult part, with both belly breathing and a dual sensory focus, is that each discipline also requires a long-term concerted effort to develop into a mental disposition that can be readily sustained, without resorting to old habits.

Our use of breathing technique though, as an effective detractor, is actually discerned from the fact that the regulating of lung fluctuations is an issue discussed by most books on resistance conditioning (or at least the ones that I have previewed). With the essence of the aforementioned practice being that we should exhale during the power stroke (or just after it) and inhale when returning the implement of impedance to its initial resting position, technically known as the eccentric contraction. All very good technique that, as a way of allowing one to excel, oftentimes becomes the basis for more effectively engaging what I of course refer to as a high-intensity specific focus. Thus explaining why, when consciously initiated, the regulating of airflow to our lungs is classified as such a potent detractor to maintaining acute muscle control.

However because of being such a compelling mechanism usually before lifting, as a way to actually clear my mind, I would concentrate specifically on controlling my breathing rhythm. Of course after grasping the implement of impedance, be it a bar or barbell, all my attention would shift to a dual sensory focus, with passive sensing engaged in discerning the subtle difference in stress between upper-arm and upper-torso control. But although no longer pursued with conscious intent the expanding and collapsing of my lungs was not completely neglected, through holding my breath. And so while lifting always remember to keep breathing, using just the movement of either arm to try and elicit a naturally syncopated rhythm.

Now the next detractor, grip tension, is actually considered a negating influence on the equilibrium effect derived from proper hand spacing. Because if the directing of the musculature of our upper-torso, to control either arm, is through strictly mental isolation then, as grip tension increases, we tend to more actively enable the musculature of our upper-arm, in effect switching our sense of control back to either extremity. Which is why, when doing either an overhead or over our chest pushing exercise, instead of gripping the barbell I would just rest it, cupped in the palm of each hand. And with the two pulling exercises, because of the contrary direction of the force vector, I would employ a hook-like grip that effectively restricted how much weight I could lift, through decreasing the amount of force I was able to resist (before my hands were forced open).

Now the final aspect, defined as a potential detractor, is the act of opening our elbow joint of either arm to the lockout position. For when that occurs and either arm is fully extended it places, in terms of over our chest and overhead pushing, each defining arm bone (on either side of each elbow joint) in a straight line to bear all the weight being lifted. And so on a conscious level, from locking-out our elbow joint, the effect is that we lose our perception of the prevailing impedance, with normally engaged muscles and tendons now offering only minimal static stability bracing. Which is not the case at every other position of either elbow joint where, within supporting muscles and tendons, an array of neural transducers usually give a more realistic indication as to the actual amount of incurred structural stress. And so along with increased grip tension extending our elbow to the point of "free" support usually signifies, in terms of sensory enhancing, that too much weight is being used.

But although defined by me as detractors of an internal nature, in terms of overcoming a set impedance, each of the three attributes just discussed is actually considered to be more facilitative in nature, as all three are usually employed to help us lift more weight. Which is of course the underlying reason why breathing, grip tension and joint locking were singled out as potential "catalysts" that can be used to direct our mindset, either towards maintaining acute muscle control by *not* taking advantage of the increased capacity each aspect is capable of eliciting. Or through our embracing of any one to all three attributes (breathing, grip tension and joint locking) to inevitably get to a point where the incurring of an injury is unfortunately what oftentimes establishes the attending limit, on the ability of our body to readily adapt.

The key though to readily acquiring the benefits, from the practicing of any type of sensory enhancing technique, is of course through just being able to maintain our focus and not get distracted. But even if seemingly a simple enough notion the actual task of not losing our concentration is however made more difficult by the fact that the only free time available, for a majority of those who are employed, is after a full day of engaging in primarily some form of mental activity. Therefore I advocate, if one has the time, working-out in the morning before having to endure a long day on the job. However since that is seldom seen as a viable option I propose (after a full day at work) taking a nap, before engaging in *any* type of sensory enhancing activity.

Finally then after completing my sensory enhancing routine to conform to my standard of a basic but thorough fitness program I would also do, usually on an inclined board, a solitary set of about twenty-five sit-ups. Where compared to the more commonly employed three sets of ten repetitions, for developing strength, a single extended set additionally encompasses improving on the stamina of my abdominal muscles, thus complementing the static endurance workout my lower-back muscles get from running and lifting weights.

That concludes my detailing of a concise resistance-conditioning program whose routine can be used as merely a series of physical exercises, for complete upper-body toning. Or through our engaging of a dual sensory focus the four lifting motions are additionally employed as a mental activity, with the added benefit of improving on the incisiveness of our initiating. Now in terms of any activity, usually employed for just extending on our ability physically excel, my use of a dual or differentiating sensory mindset, while weightlifting, was not my first attempt at consciously invoking an increase in the acuity of my spatial discerning. Because for many years already my inclination was to engage, during the early part of any extended running that I did, what can be described an aerobic sensory focus. The first half of the ensuing chapter is then about the sustaining of acute muscle control as a way to further excel when partaking in any aerobic activity although, due to my extensive experience, I have primarily considered just running.

Chapter 4

Aerobic Conditioning

Now although on a merely rudimentary level, through simply trying to improve on my overall degree of physical coordination, as a child I had oftentimes invoked an increase in the incisiveness of my initiating. What could then be called my first concerted effort at engaging a sensory focus, to specifically develop a particular motion sequence, was when I started taking tennis seriously at about the age of fourteen. In terms of strictly physical conditioning activities however my initial conscious maintaining of acute muscle control was at the age of nineteen when I first employed an aerobic sensory focus, directed at controlling how my feet made contact with the ground. Because when traversing at a leisurely gait our footfalls don't always adhere to the heel-to-toe rolling motion which, for most of us, occurs instinctively when running at a much faster pace. Instead through ignoring the muscles below our knees we tend to lazily "plop" our feet down when ambling along at the slower tempo usually employed for improving on our aerobic capacity. The concern then being that this type of casual jogging, usually exacerbated by fatigue, is oftentimes more physically stressful on the affected joints of our body compared to running at a much faster pace, which naturally creates a more fluid repetitious motion. And so as directed at maintaining a smooth heel-to-toe rolling motion the sensory focus employed, when I first started running, was simply as a way to reduce the force of impact, as caused by the act of controlled falling over an extended period of time.

About four years later, after signing up for a ten-kilometer race, is when I initially endeavored to essentially refine my aerobic sensory focus. As that entry marked the beginning of my brief interlude, into the world of competitive long-distance racing, where my insatiable curiosity was now directed at finding ways of running faster. With the result being that during early to the mid-nineteen eighties, when I ran competitively, my sustaining of acute muscle control gradually evolved as a way of more readily invoking a more rhythmic or "flowing" repetitious motion. Although even with this mental enhancement supplementing all the pre-race training I endeavored to partake in, to improve on my aerobic capacity, I was never really able to achieve anything of note, in terms of being a top finisher. However over the five years that I ran competitively, from engaging an aerobic sensory focus, I was able to steadily improve on my personal best in the 10K.

And so when there finally was an abating in my competitive fervor, since an ability to endure was still a priority with me, I continued to employ my redefined aerobic sensory focus during the early part of every fitness conditioning run I endeavored to partake in, even if eventually it would also be forsaken. Now however, as when I first started running, the shift in disposition being back to a general mindset, with more of an ignoring of inner sensory feedback, rather than a high-intensity specific focus, where a concerted effort is made at sensory suppressing. Although for a part of every run I would inevitably be compelled into invoking a sensory moderating mindset when attempting to set a faster pace or preferably, from traversing an incline, by increasing my degree of effort through an augmenting in resistance to motion. However as a result of not being as aggressive, as when racing, I was oftentimes able to engage a sensory focus long enough so that muscle counter-tension, the inherent impediment to efficient movement, was reduced to a point where there was almost a sense of effortlessness to my running.

Now integral to the actual control of any attached appendage the concept of muscle counter-tension is derived from the fact that any contorting we initiate can not only be neutralized, through a complete cessation of all movement, as it also possible to invoke a complete reversal of motion. And so muscle counter-tension is then simply a reflection of the impact of the contrary muscle group, on the motion being compelled, whenever extending or retracting some part of our body. For any movement we initiate is in fact denoted by the interacting of at least two antagonistic sets of skeletal musculature, actually working together to implement the contortion being compelled. Thus exposing acute muscle control to being merely an enhancing in our ability to not only readily direct the prime mover employed, while actively flexing some part of our body, but also the associated skeletal musculature, which opposes the motion being performed.

And while the contrary nature of a sensory focus, to maintain acute muscle control, does allow for the meticulous directing of any combination of our body's four main appendages generally though, as the example with tiptoeing demonstrated, it is not the easiest way of getting around. For by concurrently engaging both opposing sets of skeletal musculature, which primarily direct any flexing of our legs, a great deal of energy is expended on just overcoming muscle antagonism, thereby making our usual mode of locomotion less efficient. Which doesn't mean acute muscle control is never consciously maintained for an extended period of time, as ballet is probably the most graceful example of an activity that almost continuously employs this highly conflicting form of deliberately initiating the contorting of our body. If however our aim is to optimize the efficiency of any one of our various modes of transiting then, because of its inherent antagonism, our meticulous implementing of movement by traditional acute muscle control must be forsaken. For by reducing any unnecessary tensing by the associated skeletal musculature, which opposes the prime mover initiating movement, that translates into a higher percentage of contractile force actually affecting the physical displacing of some part of our body. Additionally this suppressed activity means energy is conserved by the contrary muscle group, until finally having to contract; thereby completing a return cycle of the recurring motion commonly employed by many types of physical locomotion, either real or simulated.

So what at first was defined as a counter-tension now becomes the active force, for compelling movement in the opposite direction. With walking or running this shifting in the prime mover employed actually translates into our quadriceps, initially engaged for pushing-out, needing to be relaxed as any prolonged contracting causes an increase in the amount of force needed to conduct the pulling-in motion, controlled by our hamstring muscle group. Based then on this concept of opposing forces, on which our body's lever system operates, is what fostered the idea that to develop a more rhythmic or flowing motion entailed not only controlling the specific sets of skeletal musculature engaged in initiating movement, as it also encompasses relaxing the attending muscle groups of a contrary disposition.

But although denoted primarily by the precise activating and moderating of our quadriceps and hamstrings the activity of either walking or running is also dependent on the various sets of skeletal musculature situated below our knees, which we usually tend to ignore. And so the actual refining of my original aerobic sensory focus was through extending my use of passive sensing to perceive any counter-tension being generated, by the musculature of either lower extremity. As that allowed for the invoking of a "relaxation element" which oftentimes altered, at least in a partially beneficial way, the efferent control signals for directing the specific sets of skeletal musculature which in fact control how my feet make contact with the ground.

Now when we are able to completely mitigate all unnecessary muscle counter-tension and move with the synchronicity of perfect timing, which I found relatively rare, our mental disposition also tends to become rather profound. But although having experienced, as precipitated by seemingly effortless movement, what I believe to be an elevated state of consciousness it was a book called *Flow* that really brought the concept to my attention. The reason then for not further delving into the details of my personal encounters, with this phenomenon called "flow", is because the aforementioned book already explains the concept quite thoroughly. Although in that book the notion of optimal performance was actually taken beyond fitness to the extent of being applied to other everyday activities such as work, which I could also relate to. It was then from reading about the description of such an abstract mental construct, as the various ways in which flow can be experienced, that had me once again thinking about writing a book to explain my sensory approach to resistance conditioning. The first time of course being, about five years earlier, when I initially discovered the benefits of engaging a dual sensory focus. But even after all that time, while actively practicing my mental technique, I still wasn't up to the task of putting my thoughts down on paper, so to speak.

One reason then for specifically discussing running, compared to such activities as cycling or swimming, is because developing a smooth rhythmic motion is much more demanding, when engaged in the act of controlled falling. Besides that I have been actively involved in running for over twenty years, which I can't say for cycling or swimming although I have also pursued both activities for extended periods of time. A noteworthy revelation however, from all that crossing-training experience, being the realization that, regardless of the activity I happen to be engaged in, my primary focus has really been very similar. Since ultimately whether cycling, running or swimming my overall intent has always been the same in trying to invoke a state of mind where there is a decrease in my perception of intensity, with no related diminishing in how much physical effort I am actually exerting.

A striving for effortless movement, and so not limiting my goal to being merely the completion of a set time or distance, is then the alluring psychological incentive that, even after a quarter century, has kept me intent on maintaining my aerobic capacity, through some type of physical activity. The underlying reason however, why I feel I am still able to run at my age, is because of having constrained my fitness aspirations (for the most part) to just doing what is essentially required, thereby keeping the detrimental effects of physical stress to a minimum. Also compared to ambling along at a slower set pace, for a longer period of time, my belief being that a more effective way of improving on aerobic capacity is through an activity of shorter duration but heightened intensity. With that presumption, about impacting on our body's adaptation response, being based on both the results of testing, per the law of diminishing returns, and augmented by an understanding of the various ways of harnessing cellular energy that ultimately provide the impetus, which allows for the contracting of our skeletal musculature. Because muscular activity in general, for compelling any contorting of our body, is defined by not just a single process, which releases potential energy. For any movement we initiate, through the contracting of our skeletal musculature, can in fact be compelled by at least four distinct means of metabolizing the foodstuff that we consume. And so it is not just the actual muscle fibers employed, in initiating any movement of our body, that are primarily effected, from a fairly consistent routine of some form of aerobic exercise. Because also significantly affected, from engaging in any type of activity for improving on our ability to endure, are the various energy systems of our skeletal musculature which ultimately provide the driving force that allows for varying the interlacing displacement between the micro-filaments of actin and myosin. With the term "aerobic" in fact defining two of the four forms of catabolism that although both rely on oxygen, as the impetus to compel cellular respiration, each primarily combusts just one (either fats or carbohydrates) of the two food groups usually consumed as a source of fuel. The alternative to either direct form of cellular respiration then being any energy liberating process, occurring within our cells, that doesn't require (as an intermediary) the energizing force of oxygen. And although also defined by a single term our muscles can again employ two distinct means of metabolizing the foodstuff that we consume, which in this case are anaerobic in nature.

Now with at least three of the four means of liberating cellular energy being relatively active, throughout most of our range of effort, that implies any labeling of an activity as either strictly aerobic or anaerobic can be a bit misleading. However since a physiological elucidation would require some detailing oftentimes it is just the first two related attributes of intensity and duration that are initially employed to establish where the difference lies, between what would be considered a mainly aerobic and a primarily anaerobic activity. And so from either the continuous or semi-continuous use of any number of skeletal muscle groups, to induce the complex physiological adaptations reflected superficially through simply an augmenting in our ability to endure, the degree of effort (defined as a certain target heart-rate range) must be maintained for at least ten minutes. Leading up to ten minutes then any type of moderate activity has a significant effect, in terms of inducing some sort of adaptation response. After a certain point however, with about thirty minutes being the outer limit, the benefits of exercising gradually lessen, as defined by the concept of diminishing returns. Of course what actually denotes when that drop-off occurs, in affecting an adaptation response, being our perceived degree of physical effort or intensity, as related to the particular activity we happen to be engaged in. Although through what is referred to as the principle of specific adaptation to induced demands (or SAID for short) an oftentimes significant benefit of exercising for over thirty minutes is to improve on our ability to engage in said activity, for an extended period of time. And so if the cost, in terms of wear and tear, can be kept to a minimum then working out for extended periods of time would be one way to excel at a particular activity. This practice of protracting activity length is then a viable option for both cycling and swimming where, through employing a smooth cyclical motion, physical stress is not a significant factor, although overuse is now an issue of concern. With running on the other hand, due to the more deleterious nature of the physical stress incurred, the extending of duration is a more problematic affair since similar gains in oxygen uptake, the measure of aerobic fitness, can be achieved through employing a faster pace and/or increased resistance, while keeping the actual time spent active to a minimum.

Of all the physiological adaptations incurred however, from any activity for improving on the extent of our physical stamina, the localized impact conferred on our intermediary (aerobic and anaerobic) energy systems is not the more noted or measured. For that distinction goes to our heart and lungs where, in a somewhat contrasting manner, aerobic fitness can be quantified through either the incurred decrease, in our heart rate, or as a measure of the increase in the amount of oxygen our lungs a are able to process. Although along with an augmenting in the capacity of our cardiorespiratory system research has also shown that, from participating in a routine of regular aerobic exercise, many other beneficial adaptations are incurred, although assessing the actual degree of impact is a more involved process. Leading to my belief in aerobic exercise as a wonder drug that requires at least fifteen minutes of moderate activity (to theoretically swallow) and must be taken (done) at least three times a week, for it to have a significant effect.

Now as either strictly cellular respiration or defining an anaerobic extension the underlying connection between each aforementioned metabolic process is that, although each in a different way, they all have the same ultimate purpose of recycling the actual "fuel", whose impetus allows for the contracting of our skeletal musculature. Chemically that energy source or fuel takes the form of a complex molecule known as adenosine triphosphate or ATP which, as the driving force behind a variety cellular reactions, releases energy through the detaching of a phosphate component, thereby being converted into adenosine diphosphate or ADP. Unfortunately ADP is no longer a viable energy source for powering muscle contractions or anything else, with only two phosphate attachments. Which is where each metabolic process, either extending from or directly reflecting cellular respiration, comes into the picture and creates new high-energy ATP, through expending energy reattaching free phosphate molecules to otherwise depleted molecules of ADP. And with our escalating sense of intensity, from any physical activity, being in fact denoted physiologically through a shifting in the predominant process being employed, to convert ADP back into ATP. Where with any kind of physical effort of a nominal degree of perceived intensity usually there is enough oxygen to go around and so muscle activity can be sustained through primarily direct forms of cellular respiration. As our heart starts to consume more oxygen however, from any augmenting in workload, our muscles are forced into increasingly employing other means to recycle ADP, which are more anaerobic in nature.

Ultimately though the energy we require, to engage in any type of physical activity, is initially derived from any foodstuff that we consume, which has at least some caloric content. Now between lipids and carbohydrates, the two food groups ingested primarily as a source of fuel, because at nine cal/gram it contains more than twice the potential energy of sugar, at four cal/gram, the bulk of our long-term energy requirements are normally provided for by fat. But although a more enduring process even with intense training this type of cellular respiration, which consumes primarily fat, is still too slow (in terms of recycling ADP) to meet the demands of either the fleeting or forceful motions, which our body was also designed to perform. And so to compensate for that limitation of our more enduring form of cellular respiration our muscles are able to employ not one but three additional ways that, albeit more transient, are much faster at reconverting ADP back into ATP; thus accommodating (at least to a degree) the increased demand for energy, precipitated by any sudden augmenting in our workload.

Our most expeditious metabolic process, which initially reacts to an increase in muscle activity, is then an anaerobic extension on cellular respiration based solely on high-energy molecules called creatine phosphate (CP). Essentially what happens here is (with a little enzymatic prodding) a large number of CP molecules are each induced into releasing their phosphate attachment, thereby allowing an equivalent number of depleted ADP molecules to be "recharged". An all-out physical effort however, which would be powered primarily by the breakdown of creatine phosphate, can only be sustained for about three to five seconds. Although in weightlifting this constraint on our ability to endure is actually defined through a balance between intensity and duration where, because of the disassociation of creatine phosphate (CP) occurring at a faster rate, the higher the resistance the fewer the number of repetitions possible. After a defined interval of recovery however, if not too overcome by fatigue, we are oftentimes able to perform several sets or intervals, depending on the type of strenuous activity engaged in. Of course the length of time we are able to partake in any kind of extreme physical effort is still limited, for although more persistent our other forms of cellular catabolism can never fully supplant the initial response of creatine phosphorylation.

Now if the intensity of an activity is scaled back just a little, from an all out effort, our muscles are able to employ not one but two forms of harnessing cellular energy, related to the recycling of ATP, that are in fact a reflection of the possible alternatives from a single fundamental process, the difference being in the utilization of oxygen. Of the two though, after exercising for a while, the anaerobic recycling of ADP is usually the more prolific, since an ability to operate without the impetus of oxygen makes it a more durable metabolic process. But as either direct cellular respiration or employing its anaerobic extension the underlying connection being that each is seen as essentially the "burning" of sugar to release energy, which allows for the reattaching of free phosphate fragments to expended molecules of ADP. With no oxygen however only a partial breakdown of glucose is possible and so instead of carbonic acid the anaerobic catabolism of sugar creates a secondary byproduct called lactic acid. The problem though with any acid (lactic or carbonic) is that it tends to affect a drop in the pH level of the associated intercellular solution, through accumulating faster than it can be removed. This increased acidity, as a byproduct of ATP regeneration, is then perceived as physical movement (if not curtailed) being reduced to an unrelenting sensation of physical pain. And so depending on the activity, a conditioned athlete is able to maintain a sustained level of exertion, ranging from several seconds to a few minutes, before a rather decisive impairing of physical effort, from primarily the buildup of lactic acid.

However because of not being reduced to water and carbon dioxide, the two essential building-block molecules defining the more complex structure of all fats and sugars, in effect that means lactic acid is still a viable energy source. And so rather than being simply disposed of lactic acid is instead used as a kind of kindling for continually stoking the fire of our body's long-term aerobic recycling process, which occurs in special organelles called mitochondria. Leading to the contention that, as brought on by the extended contracting of our skeletal musculature, our sense of the incurred physical stress is in part based on the fact that the ongoing anaerobic catabolism of sugar creates more lactic acid, than currently active mitochondria are able to readily "consume". Lactic acid is then envisioned as not just a trigger to activate but also as a long-term mechanism that, through our body's adaptation response, acts to impact on the number or density of muscle mitochondria. For the end result, from engaging in some form regular aerobic exercise, being that the musculature employed are compelled into creating a mitochondria reserve that is not fully enabled most of the time, since it is not needed at the relatively sedate pace at which we as normally move about. Our aerobic reserve, if we have one, would only begin to fully activate when, from a sustained level of physical activity, an increase in the anaerobic catabolism of glucose starts to create more lactic acid than currently active mitochondria are able to readily "consume". But because the breakdown of fat is a complex chemical process several minutes are required, after initially increasing our workload, for us to actually derive any benefit, from engaging our mitochondria reserve. And so what allows us to engage in events, ranging from simple quickness to sheer brute strength, is in addition to our more enduring aerobic system having a number of other ways to recycle ADP, which are not primarily dependant on oxygen. For without any anaerobic extensions on cellular respiration in theory we wouldn't be able to move very fast or lift anything heavy because, although more persistent, our aerobic regenerating of ATP could never meet the abrupt increase in demand for energy, precipitated by any sudden augmenting in our degree physical effort.

If not too overly strenuous however, after about five to seven minutes of sustained effort, what will oftentimes happen is that our perception of exertion will tend to decrease, although not from a reduction in workload. Because through an augmenting in consumption by our acquired aerobic reserve this resurgence in vigor, commonly referred to as our second wind, is in fact a reflection of a lowering in the concentration of lactic acid in the intercellular solution of the associated musculature. And so in terms of engaging an extension on cellular respiration almost every physical activity, perceived as moderately strenuous, starts out predominately anaerobic, even exercises labeled specifically as aerobic. The difference being that while for a sedentary individual the sense of effort, from a given workload, tends to rather expeditiously evolve into an overly acute sensation commonly referred to as physical pain. A more conditioned athlete is able to maintain the same set pace, at a lower perceived intensity, which readily allows his or her mitochondria reserve to fully activate in five to seven minutes and so not be subject to any impeding of effort, due a buildup of lactic acid.

But although mitochondria consume significant quantities of lactic acid these cellular organelles, as the basis to long-term cellular respiration, mainly burn fat to provide the energy needed for converting ADP back into ATP. The availability of lipids, as an energy source, is then what in fact allows for our engaging in physically demanding activities of extended duration, due to the rather insignificant persistence of even our more enduring glucose-based form of cellular respiration. And with so many people in the West, having such an ample supply of adipose tissue, it would seem an ideal group for developing extreme endurance athletes. However with always the need for at least some lactic acid, as a primer to long-term cellular respiration, that means the extent of our ability to endure is actually limited to the availability of glucose and not just having an adequate adipose reserve. With the term "hitting the wall" referring literally to the point, during a marathon or any type of extreme endurance activity, when the supply of glycogen or stored glucose (throughout our body) is almost completely used up, although fat is still readily available as source of energy. At that crucial stage what allows us to further extend our participation, instead of being forced to stop, is by our body shifting to catabolizing muscle tissue, usually from our upper-body. Since the resulting protein strands, from this dissociating of muscle tissue, are conveyed to our liver for conversion into a sugar replacement by removing any nitrogen attachments, structurally the difference between a carbohydrate and a protein. Excess nitrogen is then expelled through our urine where its concentration is usually an indicator of how ingested protein is being employed, as an amino acid building block or an energy source.

However because of being so pervasive, since we have so much muscle tissue, in effect that means the associated cellular organelles of mitochondria are then what normally constitute our primary mechanism for burning fat. Although of all the energy harnessed, through the chemical breakdown of lipids by muscular mitochondria, most of it usually derived from partaking in physical activities of low-intensity, such as when simply moving about, and not while actually exercising. And so in terms of strictly weight control, from the aerobic activity engaged in as a form of physical exercise, the primary objective shouldn't be merely an attempt to burn as many calories, at the most prodigious rate possible. For all that is really required, from the physical stress incurred, is that it compel an increase in the proliferation of muscle mitochondria, thereby affecting a discernible shift in cellular respiration to increasingly employing adipose tissue as a primary source of energy.

The question then being how to most effectively invoke this adaptation response of increasing our body's use of lipids, in the regeneration of ATP. Which is of course where the three fitness factors of intensity, duration and frequency come into play in establishing the actual constraints on some sort of exercise routine, for improving on our aerobic capacity. The problem though being that while duration and frequency fairly easy parameters to define our perception of intensity is a rather subjective sensation, dependent primarily on our prevailing state of fitness. Extensive testing however has shown that the number of beats per minute, as registered by our heart, can be a fairly impartial gauge, as to defining a set degree of effort, regardless of our current state of fitness. Although not everyone is able to denote, with a fair degree of accuracy, a set level of physical intensity, from simply referring to a chart stipulating a specific heart rate range. For what limits this concept of correlating physical effort to heart rate is that the parameters employed are generally related to the circulatory system of an average person, which only represents about eighty-percent of the population (in terms of a bell curve). But since the other twenty-percent, whose heart size doesn't conform to the norm, are not readily identified to establish if the degree of physical effort is sufficient the old-fashioned method of employing passive sensing, as simply an intensity gauge, should not be forsaken.

That then completes a rather superficial description of a thorough, albeit sparse, fitness conditioning routine where nothing I have said is really new, in terms of the augmenting in strength and stamina that can be acquired. What makes my approach unique is of extending to incorporate the sustaining of acute muscle control, as expressed through either a dual sensory mindset (with resistance conditioning) or an aerobic sensory focus (when running). In the final chapter however a sensory approach to fitness is viewed in terms of its related psychological benefit, which many have claimed they derived from partaking in some sort of physical activity. Although my underlying intent is to expose a possible detriment to limiting our outlook to either the more relaxed disposition of a general mindset or, at the other extreme of the fitness spectrum, the overly competitive demeanor of a high-intensity specific focus.

Chapter 5

Sensory Input

Now in considering the physiological basis to a psychological benefit, from most any type of physical activity, a comparative analogy will again be made. Although instead of sensory information processing being described in terms of serial or parallel, as with a computer, the structuring of our brain is compared to how a radio or television receiver operates. For like a variety of electronic devices (of which the more obvious examples being radio and television) our neural processing system can only "tune in" and process a set amount of sensory information, from the total bandwidth transmitted by our five senses. However unlike the very narrow frequency spectrum employed for detecting a single a radio or television station, our brain is able to decode and analyze a much wider bandwidth of sensory information. As normally each sense contributes a certain amount of input to the summation of sensations, which we define as our perceived reality.

In today's high-tech world however, as defined by the amount of sensory stimuli we subject ourselves to, it would seem that our eyes and ears have encroached on a better part of that spectrum of sensory information flowing to our brain although what our other senses contribute, especially our sense of touch, is obviously as important if not more so. With the contention being that the transmission bandwidth allocated to each sense is a significant factor in affecting how we perceive ourselves as a physical entity. For example if the channel for processing auditory sensory information was "wider" than normal that would translate into an inherent ability to more intricately analyze sound; thereby underlying the premise proposing the notion of a disposition towards music, based on strictly genetics. An increase in auditory processing bandwidth could however also be incurred through nurturing, if we just happened to like and therefore spend a lot of time listening to music. Now should there be a sudden diminishing in our augmented sense of hearing, for whatever reason, naturally our perception of reality would be severely impaired and probably require an extended period of psychological reconciling, to regain a semblance of normality.

Going deaf or blind is however a more perceptible loss of allotted bandwidth, for the processing of sensory information; less detectable, although probably no less deleterious, is when a diminishing in our sense of touch takes place. Now the basis for that presumption (on the importance of our sense of touch) seems rather obvious as related to the more perceptible interface between our brain and our body. What I am alluding to is the more elusive connection between neural sensory information and its underlying effect on our mind. For the importance of sensory stimuli beyond its strictly tangible association was first noted, with scientific scrutiny, during sensory deprivation experiments that, as an expressed form of mental instability, induced hallucinations. Although it was only when, along with blocking both visual and auditory stimuli, our sense of touch was also repressed that, by their own account, a significant number of those tested readily experienced this psyche unbalancing, manifested as visual delusions. Hence my contention that through defining our physical presence in the world an important attribute of our sense of touch, both inner and outer, is as a stabilizing influence on our mental psyche, thus defining its psychological significance.

The concern then being that, although made for just stimulating our eyes and ears, one of today's most ubiquitous technological marvels is also indirectly employed in deleteriously impacting on the stabilizing influence conveyed by our sense of touch. Not through sensory depravation however, although sitting motionless for hours could be a factor, but by diminishing the bandwidth segment for the processing of sensory information from both our inner and outer sense of touch. Because although it would appear that the total spectrum of our conscious awareness is seemingly variable in size; it is also likely that there is a limit where excessive stimulation, in this case to both our eyes and ears, results in reducing the amount of sensory information that our other three senses are able to get through. And so on a conscious level, from mainly watching television, an augmenting in both audio and visual processing would then be reflected not only through a diminishing in our sense of touch, but also by a moderating in the sensitivity of both our sense of smell and taste. Although if perceived, because we use some type of odor masking, our reaction to a slight dulling in smell sensitivity would probably be limited to simply applying a higher concentration of fragrance. And with a decrease in our sense of taste, which may be more obvious, our response would likely be confined to just adding more flavor enhancer (usually sugar or salt) to the food we eat. Now with our sense of touch both attributes have been considered, the physical and the psychological, because of each one usually being more profound than with either our sense of smell or taste, where only the more tangible aspect has been taken into account. And so the more discernable effect of a slight moderating in the acuity of our sense of touch would then be perceived as merely an increased tolerance to all types of physical pain. While the more abstract psychological consequence is expressed, in terms of self-awareness, as an invoked diminishing in our sensing of our physical presence.

Now if by chance this tempering of how we perceive our tangible self somehow becomes an issue, through whatever means, it can create a sense of such import as to actually trigger a quest to somehow find a way of revitalizing that diminished aspect, which gives stability to our mental psyche. For some a resolution is seemingly achieved with a quick-fix solution, usually through an activity that employs fear as a mechanism to suddenly traumatize one into feeling more "alive". Others less adventurous, as a way to create a uniqueness to one's presence that isn't felt, may simply resort to changing the way they look, from just dressing differently to more enduring forms of body art or mutilation (depending on one's point view). But as caused by the encroaching of an expanding bandwidth, from high levels of stimulation to both our eyes and ears, how can this repressing of our sense of touch be curtailed, with the process even possibly being reversed?

Well that is where my other evidence on the importance of our sense of touch comes from. For as it revitalized not only the author's body but also strengthened his or her mental psyche a number of publications have addressed the idea that the invigorating stimulation, from almost any type of physical activity, also included a psychological aspect. Notable among these writers being the late Dr. George Sheehan who, throughout his writing, essentially elaborated on what he felt was a lack of an appreciation for all the mental benefits incurred, from simply being physically active. With regards to sports however the problem of course being that most of us are spectators, not participants, and of the few who do happen to play the obsession appears to be with quantifying every aspect, with no reflection on the sheer joy of being physically active. As for those who do exercise, just for the health of it, most seem to regard inner sensory feedback as simply physical pain; consequently something to be ignored through being distracted by some other mental activity, such as interfacing with a media device or simply reading. Leading to my contention that Tai Chi and Yoga are two of a scant number of explicit disciplines that, through their invoking of an increase in the acuity of our spatial discerning, directly augment the psychological stabilizing influence conveyed by our inner sense of touch.

Of course through the practicing of any series of concise motions, such as with dancing or any other exacting competitive activity, it is also possible to improve on our degree of kinesthetic awareness. Oftentimes though visual feedback can actually act as a subtle detractor, when reiterating some aspect of our sport of choice (especially when our attention is not directed at the contortion being performed but merely its resulting consequence, as for example where the ball lands). And as for dancing its rejuvenating quality is oftentimes deleteriously impacted on from simultaneously being exposed to high levels of competing forms of sensory stimulation, in this case bright lights and loud music. Leading to my contention that engaging a dual or differentiating sensory focus, when weightlifting, is then one way to extend on the possible constraints of either type of activity, for improving on the incisiveness of our initiating. Additionally of course, through maintaining acute muscle control, a dual sensory approach also encompasses the psychological benefit incurred from the practice of Tai Chi and similar disciplines where, from simply invoking an increase in the acuity of our spatial discerning, there is an enhancing in the connection between body and mind.

Naturally there are advantages to having a wider transmission bandwidth for the increased processing of both auditory and visual information. Otherwise music videos (because of a propensity for scene shifting) would be very disorienting and rap music (because of the pace at which the verbalizations are delivered) would be impossible to understand. One possible reason then why so many baby boomers and beyond don't really care either form of musical expression, videos or rap, is because of their mental faculties not initially being attuned to processing such a high rate of information. As alluded to however there are also possibly related psychological detriments, associated with having an overly augmented ability at both audio and visual processing. With one concern being that, as defined through just physical appearance or what people say, our sense of self-worth shifts to being very superficially based on merely external stimuli. But defined by me as simply invoking an enhanced sense of our physical presence it still took some time for me to assess the significance of how it all related to a dual sensory approach. And so the question is how can the mental benefits incurred, from any physical activity, be readily "quantified" in such a way that actually allows for some type of objective determination to be made. Or does this delving into the psychological impact of physical exercise have to wait for a more thorough understanding of the exact nature of that seemingly differentiated entity usually referred to as simply our mind?

And so through a functional embodying of our sense of self-awareness, as defined by the bilateral structure of our brain, that concludes my dissertation defining how to improve on the incisiveness of our initiating. And while probably not furthering the field of neuroscience my detailing should have allowed for at least a working understanding of how to effectively engage a dual sensory focus, to extend the benefits incurred beyond the strictly physical.